Teaching Cultural Competence in Nursing and Health Care

About the Author

Marianne R. Jeffreys EdD, RN, received a BS in nursing from the State University of New York College at Plattsburgh; an MA and MEd in nursing education/professorial role from Teachers College, Columbia University; and an EdD in nursing education/nurse executive from Teachers College, Columbia University. She is a member of Kappa Delta Pi International Honor Society in Education (Columbia University Chapter) and a member of Sigma Theta Tau International Honor Society in Nursing (Mu Upsilon Chapter). An international award recipient, Dr. Jeffreys received the 2003 Leininger Award for Excellence in Transcultural Nursing from the Transcultural Nursing Society. Currently a professor at the City University of New York College of Staten Island, her teaching experience with diverse student populations includes medical-surgical nursing, nursing research, and transcultural nursing at the associate baccalaureate, and master's degree levels. Her grant-funded research, consultations, publications, and professional presentations encompass the topics of transcultural nursing, nontraditional nursing students, student retention and achievement, self-efficacy, teaching, curriculum, and psychometrics. Dr. Jeffreys is also the author of *Nursing Student Retention: Understanding the Process and Making a Difference.*

Teaching Cultural Competence in Nursing and Health Care:

Inquiry, Action, and Innovation

Marianne R. Jeffreys, EdD, RN

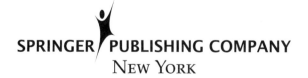

SPRINGER PUBLISHING COMPANY
New York

Springer Publishing Company, Inc.
11 West 42nd Street
New York, NY 10036

Acquisitions Editor: Sally J. Barhydt
Production Editor: Judi Rohrbaugh
Cover Design: Joanne E. Honigman
Composition by TechBooks

06 07 08 09 10 / 5 4 3 2 1

Library of Congress Cataloging-in-Publication Data

Jeffreys, Marianne R. Teaching cultural competence in nursing and health care : inquiry,
    action, and innovation / Marianne R. Jeffreys.
        p. ; cm.
    Includes bibliographical references and index.
    ISBN 0-8261-7764-6 (alk. paper)
    1. Transcultural nursing. 2. Minorities—Medical care.
        3. Nursing—Social aspects, I. Title.
    [DNLM: 1. Transcultural Nursing—education. WY 18 J46: 2006]
RT86.5.J442 2006
610.73—dc22

2006011532

Printed in the United States of America by Bang Printing.

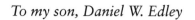

To my son, Daniel W. Edley

Contents

PART I. Tools to Get Started

PART II. Educational Activities for Easy Application

Contents

List of Figures, Tables, and Boxes

Preface

Preparing nurses and other health professionals to provide quality health care in the increasingly multicultural and global society of the 21st century requires a new, comprehensive approach that emphasizes cultural competence education throughout professional education and professional life. *Teaching Cultural Competence in Nursing and Health Care* aims to address this need and provide readers with valuable tools and strategies for cultural competence education at all levels.

Culture is a factor that can make the greatest difference in promoting wellness, preventing illness, restoring health, facilitating coping, and enhancing quality of life for all individuals, families, and communities. The two major goals of the U.S. Department of Health and Human Services report *Healthy People 2010* require culture-specific care. The first goal—to increase quality and years of healthy life for all—can only be achieved when examining "quality of life" and the meaning of "health and well-being" within a cultural context. The second goal seeks to eliminate health disparities among different segments of the population, necessitating culture-specific and competent actions designed to eliminate disparities (Jeffreys, 2005b). Therefore, customized health care that fits the client's cultural values, beliefs, and traditions (culturally congruent care) is urgently imperative (Leininger, 2002a, 2002b).

Culturally congruent health care is a basic human right, not a privilege, and therefore every human should be entitled to it. The International Council of Nurses (ICN) *Code for Nurses* (ICN, 1973), the American Nurses Association (ANA) Code of Ethics (ANA, 2001), and the *National Standards for Culturally and Linguistically Appropriate Services in Health Care* (Office of Minority Health, 2001) are several important documents that serve as reminders. Criteria within accreditation and credentialing agencies such as the Joint Commission on Accreditation of Healthcare Organizations, the National Committee on Quality

Assurance, the American Medical Association, and the National League for Nursing strive to assure that culturally competent health care services and education are provided. Not only are nurses, physicians, other health care providers, and institutions ethically and morally obligated to provide the best culturally congruent care possible, but they are also legally mandated to do so. Within the scope of professional practice, nurses and other health professionals are expected to actively seek out ways to promote culturally congruent care. Yet, providing such care to the myriad culturally diverse populations is a growing professional challenge.

Educators everywhere are additionally challenged to learn how to effectively lead the quest for culturally congruent health care by implementing creative, evidence-based educational activities that promote positive, cultural competence learning outcomes for a diverse body of students and health care professionals. Ongoing questions and requests from educators and researchers around the world, within various health disciplines, and within different settings revealed a critical gap in educational resources specifically focused on the teaching–learning process of cultural competence. Written in response to this need, this book is intended as a primary resource for educators and graduate students in academic settings, health care institutions (HCIs), and professional associations. In this book, readers will find the following resources:

- A model to guide cultural competence education
- A questionnaire for measuring and evaluating learning
- A guide for identifying at-risk individuals and avoiding pitfalls
- A wide selection of educational activities
- Techniques for diverse learners
- Vignettes, case examples, illustrations, tables, and assessment tools

This hands-on, user-friendly book is divided into two parts: Part I, Tools to Get Started, and Part II, Educational Activities for Easy Application. Part I contains four chapters filled with resources and tools to help educators begin teaching cultural competence. Essential background information about the multidimensional process of teaching cultural competence offers a valuable guide for educators at all levels when planning, implementing, and evaluating cultural competence education.

Chapter 1 begins with an overview of the key issues, concerns, and new challenges facing health care consumers, professionals, and educators today and in the future. Professional goals, societal needs, ethical considerations, legal issues, changing demographics, and learner characteristics are highlighted. Select cultural values and beliefs are vividly compared and contrasted in a supplementary table that enhances the text. The chapter concludes with a discussion of factors influencing cultural competence development among culturally diverse learners and proposes that confidence, or in the context of this book transcultural self-efficacy (TSE), is a major component in cultural competence development and a strong influencing factor in the achievement of culturally congruent care.

Chapter 2 introduces a model to guide cultural competence education—the Cultural Competence and Confidence (CCC) model. The underlying assumptions, principles, concepts, and terms associated with the model's development are concisely presented. A unique feature of the model (and the book) is that its major concepts, propositions, and constructs are supported by several quantitative studies using the questionnaire also presented in this book. The visual illustration of the model enhances understanding of the text. A second illustration expands on the CCC model illustration by tracing the proposed influences of TSE (confidence) on a learner's actions, performance, and persistence for learning tasks associated with cultural competency development and culturally congruent care. The model is brought to life through a realistic "Educator-in-Action" vignette featuring cultural competence education in the health care institution (hospital setting).

Educators and researchers are continually challenged to measure changes following educational interventions. Chapter 3 addresses this challenge by introducing a quantitative tool (questionnaire) that measures and evaluates learners' confidence—the Transcultural Self-Efficacy Tool (TSET). The TSET has been used in several grant-funded projects and studies, and has been requested by graduate students, faculty, and health care professionals in various disciplines from around the world. These ongoing requests identified the need to write this book and to provide detailed information about the TSET and the conceptual model underlying it. Major components, features, and psychometric properties (reliability and validity) of the 83-item questionnaire are presented, using a systematic and reader-friendly approach. Tables summarize vital instrument information. The TSET and accompanying appendices provide valuable resources for educational researchers. Applied uses, evaluation strategies, and the "Educator-in-Action" vignette conclude the chapter, offering multiple options and ideas for educators and researchers.

Chapter 4 offers resources for establishing prioritized, diagnostic-prescriptive, evidence-based cultural competence education. For example, inefficacious (low confidence) individuals are at risk for decreased motivation, lack of commitment, and/or avoidance of cultural considerations when planning and implementing nursing care. In addition, supremely efficacious (overly confident) individuals are at risk for inadequate preparation in learning the transcultural nursing skills necessary to provide culturally congruent care. Implications for educators are presented.

Pragmatic suggestions for avoiding pitfalls in educational research design and data interpretation are also offered. The "Educator-in-Action" vignette provides a clear example of how educators may easily integrate this guided approach within their own teaching practice.

Part II offers a wide selection of educational activities that can easily be applied by educators everywhere. Chapter 5 introduces readers to strategies aimed at uncovering, discovering, and exploring educational opportunities within academia for promoting cultural competency, beginning with faculty self-assessment. An illustrated self-assessment tool for faculty and students provides an excellent resource for easy use. Inquiry, action, and innovation at the curriculum level involve the philosophy, conceptual framework, program objectives, program outcomes, courses, course components, horizontal threads, and vertical threads. At the course level, inquiry, action, and innovation involve the course outline, instructional media, learning activities, course components, and clinical settings. Detailed examples include the teaching of cultural competence through innovative use of textbooks, reading assignments, videos, computer-assisted instruction, web page, nursing skills laboratory, clinical settings, written assignments, presentations, exams, and supplementary resources. These resources involve the library, enrichment programs, nursing student club, nursing student resource center, bulletin boards, honor society chapter, local organizations, and guest speakers. Action-focused strategies for educational innovation and ideas for evaluating educational interventions are described throughout the chapter, concluding with a descriptive "Educator-in-Action" vignette.

In Chapter 6, strategies for systematic inquiry into already existing facets of the health care institution (HCI) are proposed, along with suggested activities for developing new initiatives, actions, educational innovation, and evaluation. An illustrated self-assessment tool for direct application within HCIs, a sample questionnaire to guide prioritization, and a sample list for determining target populations are essential tools to guide cultural competence education and justify resource allocation. Numerous examples of educational activities are integrated throughout the chapter, highlighting key areas such as institutional mission and philosophy, new employee orientation, newsletter and publications, in-service education, staff meetings, patient care conferences, walking rounds and report, special events, continuing education, and networking. The "Educator-in-Action" vignette demonstrates several strategies thoughtfully integrated to maximize the vast resources of culturally diverse health professionals within a health care institution servicing many different groups of patients.

Professional associations possess a potentially powerful and extensive ability to network diverse and talented groups of professionals beyond a single health care institution or academic setting; therefore, professional associations can exert tremendous influence on promoting, disseminating, and advancing cultural competence education. Chapter 7 highlights strategies for identifying educational opportunities within professional associations for promoting cultural competence education; recognizing and overcoming barriers and challenges; and developing action-focused strategies for educational innovation. An illustrated assessment tool is provided for direct application within these associations, and numerous educational activities are presented. A thought-provoking table compares and contrasts educational topics and titles, challenging associations to go "beyond topic and title to search for substantive evidence of cultural competence." The "Educator-in-Action" vignette presents a realistic scenario that illustrates several ongoing challenges facing professional associations today.

Chapter 8 suggests important implications for educators everywhere. Educators are challenged to commit to a focused and transformational change that will not only advance the science and art of cultural competence education, but will also result in culturally congruent care, ultimately benefiting health care consumers worldwide. The urgent expansion of educational research specifically focused on the teaching and learning of cultural competence is emphasized, and areas for further inquiry, research, and future goals are proposed. Extensive references and relevant appendices are provided at the end of the book.

The ideas and suggestions presented here are not meant to be exhaustive, but are offered with the intent to stimulate new ideas and invite health professionals to explore new paths on the winding journey to developing cultural competence in oneself and in others. Readers are encouraged to pause, reflect, and question throughout the book in order to gain new insights and perspectives. Everyone is empowered to contribute to a transformational change in health care that prioritizes cultural competence development and embraces diversity.

Acknowledgments

Partial funding for previous research on the Transcultural Self-Efficacy Tool (TSET) and the assessment of students' transcultural self-efficacy perceptions was obtained from the Nursing Education Alumni Association of Teachers College, Columbia University Postdoctoral Research Fellowship Award; The Research Foundation of the City University of New York PSC-CUNY Research Award Program; The City University of New York College of Staten Island Division of Science and Technology Research Award; and the Mu Upsilon Chapter of Sigma Theta Tau International Honor Society in Nursing.

PART I

Tools to Get Started

CHAPTER 1

Overview of Key Issues and Concerns

Meeting the health care needs of culturally diverse clients has become even more challenging and complex. In addition to acknowledging the cultural evolution (growth and change) occurring in the United States (and other parts of the world), it is imperative that nursing and other health care professions appreciate and understand the impending cultural revolution. The term *cultural revolution* implies a "revolution of thinking" that seeks to embrace the evolution of a different, broader worldview (Jeffreys & Zoucha, 2001). Both cultural evolution and cultural revolution have the potential to bring about a different worldview regarding cultural care and caring by including key issues previously nonexistent, underrepresented, or invisible in the nursing and health care literature. This new vision challenges all health care professionals to embark on a new journey in the quest for cultural competence and culturally congruent care for all clients (Jeffreys & Zoucha, 2001). Educators everywhere are additionally challenged to learn how to effectively lead the quest for culturally congruent health care by implementing creative, evidence-based educational activities that promote positive, cultural competence learning outcomes for culturally diverse students and health care professionals.

This transformational journey begins by seeking to understand the key issues, concerns, and new challenges facing health care consumers and professionals today and in the future. This chapter evokes professional awareness, sparks interest, stimulates revolutionary thought, highlights vital information, and shares new ideas concerning the health care needs of culturally diverse clients and the development of cultural competence among culturally diverse health care professionals. *Cultural competence* has been described as a multidimensional process that aims to achieve culturally congruent health care (Andrews & Boyle, 2002;

3

Campinha-Bacote, 2003; Leininger, 1991a; Purnell & Paulanka, 2003). Culturally congruent health care refers to health care that is customized to fit with the client's cultural values, beliefs, traditions, practices, and lifestyle (Leininger, 1991a). It is beyond the scope of this chapter to provide a summary review of the existing literature concerning cultural competence and health care. Rather, this chapter emphasizes select points from the literature, identifies future complexities and challenges in health care, discusses factors influencing cultural competency development, and proposes a new construct involved in the process of cultural competence development and education.

COMPLEXITIES, CHANGES, AND CHALLENGES IN HEALTH CARE

Rapid growth in worldwide migration, changes in demographic patterns, varying fertility rates, increased numbers of multiracial and multiethnic individuals, and advanced technology contribute to cultural evolution. For the purpose of this book, *cultural evolution* refers to the process of cultural growth and change within a society (Jeffreys & Zoucha, 2001). Within the nursing literature, cultural growth, change, and the need for culturally congruent nursing care has been frequently reported in various countries, including Australia, Canada, Sweden, South Africa, and the United Kingdom (Davidson, Meleis, Daly, & Douglas, 2003; Douglas, 2000). Although this book addresses cultural changes in the United States, readers should recognize that globalization is a worldwide phenomenon with populations now moving more frequently than ever before. Because more people are migrating several different places, the acculturation experience may include cultural values and beliefs (CVB) assimilated from more than one source, resulting in new ways of expressing traditional CVB and/or resulting in new cultural values and belief patterns. Consequently, health care professionals are challenged to meet the needs of changing societies in new and different ways.

The 2000 U.S. Census (U.S. Census Bureau, 2002) and Healthy People 2010 (Department of Health and Human Services [DHHS], 2000) provide valuable data about select population characteristics; however, they are limited in providing information about cultural values, beliefs, behaviors, and practices associated with the many diverse cultural groups existing within the United States. For example, it is helpful to know that minority populations are increasing more rapidly than white non-Hispanic, nonimmigrant populations (as determined by such variables as age and fertility rates), further justifying and demanding increased population-specific resource allocation. It is also crucial to have identified health disparities, high priority areas, goals, and proposed strategies for improvement; however, nurses and other health care professionals must become actively aware of the diverse cultural groups comprising each designated minority category if Healthy People 2010 (DHHS, 2000) goals are to be met. For example, the "Hispanic" category may include individuals whose heritage may be traced to Cuba, Nicaragua, Mexico, Puerto Rico, Peru, Spain, and/or other countries, each also representing much diversity within and between groups. Diversity may exist based on birthplace, citizenship status, reason for migration, migration history, food, religion, ethnicity, race, language, kinship and family networks, educational background and opportunities, employment skills and opportunities, lifestyle, gender, socioeconomic status (class), politics, past discrimination and bias experiences, health status and health risk, age, insurance coverage, and other variables that go well beyond the restrictive labels of a few ethnic and/or racial groups.

The projected increase of multiracial and multiethnic (multiple heritage) individuals both in the United States (Johnson, 1997; Lee & Fernandez, 1998; Perlmann, 1997; Sands & Schuh, 2004; Spickard & Fong, 1995) and throughout the world demonstrates a growing change in demographic patterns, adding to this new cultural evolution. Forced single category choices and/or the "other" category makes the unique culture of the multiracial and multiethnic individual invisible (Jeffreys, 2005a, 2005b; Jeffreys & Zoucha, 2001). Although the 2000 U.S. Census permitted individuals to select more than one racial/ethnic category, the lateness of this option demonstrates the reluctance for society to acknowledge and appreciate the existence of mestizo (mixing) in the United States (Nash, 1995). The late repeal of the last laws against miscegenation (race mixing) in the 1970s attests not only to societal reluctance, but also to political resistance reflecting racial ideologies of some white Americans (Pascoe, 1996).

Inconsistent use of the data from individuals selecting more than one census category is confusing and typically favors the antiquated process of assigning individuals to one category only; usually, the minority status or politically advantageous category is selected. For example, when reporting the number of "minority" individuals within a public school system for the purpose of demonstrating integration within a predominantly white school, someone selecting "black" and "white" would be assigned as being "black." In reality, it may be impossible for a multiethnic and/or multiracial individual to choose one ethnic or racial identity over the other (Hall, 1992; Pinderhughes, 1995). Multiple heritage identity can include membership within one select group, simultaneous membership with two or more distinct groups, synthesis (blending) of cultures, and/or fluid identities with different groups that change with time, circumstance, and setting (Daniel, 1992; Root, 1992; Spickard & Fong, 1995). Moreover, multiple heritage individuals often describe being "multiracial" or "multiethnic" as a separate and unique culture (Root, 1997; Spickard, 1997). Culturally congruent health care for the 6,826,228 individuals who identified as being of more than one race in the 2000 U.S. Census (U.S. Census Bureau, 2002) must begin with openly acknowledging the uniqueness of multiple heritage individuals and seeking to learn about their lived experience. Multiple heritage individuals present unique concerns and challenges for transcultural nurses and other health care professionals because of the lack of research and published studies in nursing and health care (Jeffreys, 2005a, 2005b; Jeffreys & Zoucha, 2001).

Similarly, other underrepresented, invisible, unpopular, or new issues present complexities and challenges to health care professionals because of the lack of substantive research, resources, and expertise specifically targeting such topics related to culture and changing populations (cultural evolution). With the rapid changes and influx of new populations from around the world, nurses are faced with the challenge of caring for many different cultural groups than ever before. Changes are occurring more rapidly in urban, suburban, and rural areas, often with cultural groups clustering together in ethnic neighborhoods. This means that there is less time for nurses to learn about and become accustomed to new cultural groups. Lack of nurses with transcultural nursing expertise presents a severe barrier in meeting the health care needs of diverse client populations (Leininger & McFarland, 2002).

Political changes throughout the world have resulted in large migration waves from former socialist, communist, monarchy, and dictatorship nations. Too many choices (in health care planning options) may overwhelm individuals who are not used to such freedoms (Miller, 1997). Mismatches in expectations between health care professional and client can cause poor health outcomes, stress, and dissatisfaction. Nurses unfamiliar with various political systems and the potential impact on clients' perceptions may be unprepared to provide culturally congruent care for these clients. Understanding the ethnohistory, especially the influence of politics, economics, discrimination, and intergroup and intragroup conflicts, is an important cultural dimension that warrants further attention (Davidson et al., 2003; Leininger & McFarland, 2002; Miller, 1997). Despite the commonality of national origin, cultural experiences may be quite different for persons seeking asylum, refugees, and immigrants, and may vary at different points in history, necessitating an accurate and individualized appraisal.

Health care professionals are also challenged to differentiate between numerous minority groups around the world (who may have been victims of overt and/or covert stereotyping, prejudice, discrimination, and racism) and dominant groups. Within the United States, it has been well documented that discrimination, stereotyping, prejudice, and racism exist in nursing and health care (Abrums & Leppa, 2001; American Nurses Association [ANA], 1998; Barbee & Gibson, 2001; Bolton, Giger, & Georges, 2004; Farella, 2002; Porter & Barbee, 2004). This unpopular topic has not gained the sufficient attention and action necessary to actively dismantle stereotyping, prejudice, discrimination, and racism. Raising awareness is insufficient; taking appropriate and definitive action through well-planned positive innovative interventions followed by evaluation strategies will move beyond complacent "passive advocacy" to positive "active innovative advocacy." Such innovative actions require development of cultural competence and sincere commitment on the part of health care professionals.

Groups identified as "subcultures" have been identified as "vulnerable populations"; such populations present complex scenarios to health care professionals today and will do so in the future. For example, illegal immigrants, migrant workers, tenant farmers, and the homeless often present unique health care challenges due to lack of health insurance, illiteracy, poverty, and fear. In addition, tenant farmers and migrant workers may be buried together under the heading of "rural health"; thus, the truly unique culture(s) and needs within and between groups across various geographic regions may remain undiscovered. Because tenant farmers may receive food and housing as part of their wages, tenant farmers may not be eligible for food stamps; Medicaid; Women, Infants, and Children; public assistance; or other social services. Employee benefits such as health insurance and dental insurance are usually nonexistent. Funds for clothing, soap, toothpaste, toothbrushes, and other toiletries may be scarce, making tenant farmers susceptible to preventable diseases. Geographic isolation and lack of transportation are barriers encountered within rural communities, thus presenting another barrier to health care access. Within the United States, health insurance diversity presents inconsistencies in health care, especially in health promotion and illness prevention. Consequently, primary care is not routinely accessible, with delayed entry into the health care system occurring for treatment of acute and advanced problems.

Rapidly moving populations bring unfamiliar diseases, new diseases, treatments, and medicines, challenging health care professionals to become quickly proficient in accurate diagnosis, treatment, and prevention. For example, nurses unfamiliar with malaria may be suddenly faced with several refugees from Africa who require treatment for malaria. New diseases, such as severe acute respiratory syndrome, can cause epidemics if not identified early and then properly controlled. Medicines and treatments considered "alternative" or "complementary" within the culture of Western medicine may actually be considered "routine" in other cultures. Medicines considered "routine" within the culture of Western medicine may have varying and adverse effects with different ethnic or racial groups due to health beliefs and/or due to genetic differences in body processes (e.g., metabolism) and/or anatomical characteristics (e.g., sun absorption based on skin color). The growing new field of ethnopharmacology attests to the urgent need to investigate the pharmacokinetics, pharmacodynamics, and overall pharmacological effects of drugs within specific cultural groups. Unfortunately, insurance company approval for drug therapy regimen is often guided by drug studies among primarily homogeneous populations rather than taking into account new, however sparse, empirical evidence provided by ethnopharmacological studies.

Inconsistencies in the expected roles of the nurse may vary from culture to culture, therefore confounding the therapeutic nurse–client interaction, nurse–nurse interaction, nurse–physician interaction, and nurse–family interaction. Whether the nurse is viewed as a well-educated professional, vocational service provider, paraprofessional, uneducated worker, or servant will greatly impact the therapeutic and working relationship (Purnell, 2003). Furthermore, whether the nurse is viewed as an outsider, "stranger," "trusted friend," or insider will significantly influence the nurse–client relationship, the achievement of culturally congruent care, and optimal health outcomes (Leininger, 2002c). The mismatch between the diversity of registered nurses and U.S. populations presents one large barrier to meeting the needs of diverse populations. For example, white nurses of European American heritage represent approximately 90% of all registered nurses (Barbee & Gibson, 2001; Kimball & O'Neill, 2002).

Expected roles and perceptions about other health care professionals will also vary from culture to culture, thus necessitating an accurate appraisal of clients' baseline knowledge, beliefs, and expectations if culturally congruent care is to be achievable by the multidisciplinary health care team. Gender roles and expectations about members of the health care team are variable. Within certain cultures, it may be unacceptable for women to become physicians and provide care for male patients; conversely, it may be unacceptable for men to become nurses and provide care for female patients (St. Hill, Lipson, & Meleis, 2003). In some cultures there may not be a word or concept for "psychologist," "psychiatrist," "dietician," "social worker," or "recreational therapist," thus presenting new challenges for health care professionals in Western society. For example, there is no word in Korean for psychologist or psychiatrist; mental illness is highly stigmatized with clients and families encountering great difficulties when mental illness occurs (Donnelly, 1992, 2005). This requires students, nurses, the nursing profession, and other health care professionals to become active participants (and partners) in the process of developing cultural competence and to actively seek and embrace a broad (even revolutionary) worldview of diversity.

ETHICAL AND LEGAL ISSUES

Culturally congruent health care is a basic human right, not a privilege (ANA, 1991, 2001; Cameron-Traub, 2002; International Council of Nurses [ICN], 1973; Leininger, 1991a, 1991b); therefore, every human should be entitled to culturally congruent care. In addition, empirical findings clearly document the strong link between culturally congruent care and the achievement of positive health outcomes. Increasing numbers of lawsuits with clients claiming that culturally appropriate care was not rendered by hospitals, physicians, nurses, and other health care providers attest to the complicated legal issues that may arise from culturally incongruent care. Furthermore, clients are often winning their cases in court (Leininger & McFarland, 2002). The ICN *Code for Nurses* (ICN, 1973), the ANA Code of Ethics (ANA, 2001), and the *National Standards for Culturally and Linguistically Appropriate Services in Health Care* (Office of Minority Health [OMH], 2001) are several important documents that serve as reminders and provide guidance to health professionals. Not only are nurses and other health care providers ethically and morally obligated to provide the best culturally congruent care possible, but also they are legally mandated to do so. Within the scope of professional practice, nurses and other health professionals are expected to actively seek out ways to promote culturally congruent care.

To "assist, support, facilitate, or enhance" culturally congruent care, Leininger (1991a) proposed three modes for guiding nursing decision and actions: (a) cultural care preservation and/or maintenance, (b) culture care accommodation and/or negotiation, and (c) culture care repatterning and/or restructuring. Because culturally congruent care can only occur when culture care values, expressions, or patterns are known and used appropriately (Leininger, 1995a), a systematic, thorough cultural assessment is a necessary precursor to planning and implementing care (Andrews & Boyle, 2002; Campinha-Bacote, 2003; Giger & Davidhizar, 1999; Leininger, 2002a, 2002c; Purnell & Paulanka, 2003; Spector, 2004). Assessment, planning, implementing, and evaluating culturally congruent care requires active, ongoing learning based on theoretical support and empirical evidence. The goal of culturally congruent care can only be achieved through the process of developing (learning and teaching) cultural competence (Jeffreys, 2006).

BARRIERS

Professional goals, societal needs, ethical considerations, and legal issues all declare the need to prioritize cultural competence development, necessitating a conscious, committed, and transformational change in current nursing practice, education, and research (Jeffreys, 2002). Although nursing can be transformed through the teaching of transcultural nursing (Andrews, 1995; Leininger, 1995a, 1995b; Leininger & McFarland, 2002), two major barriers prevent a rapid effective transformation. One major barrier is the lack of faculty and advanced practice nurses formally prepared in transcultural nursing and in the teaching of transcultural nursing (Andrews, 1995; Jeffreys, 2002; Leininger, 1995b). The second major barrier is the limited research evaluating the effectiveness of teaching interventions on the development of cultural competence (Jeffreys, 2002). These two barriers are further complicated by the (a) changing demographics of students and health care professionals and (b) severe shortage of nurses and nursing faculty. Several of these factors are highlighted in the following sections. Part II of this book presents action strategies, innovations, and practical examples for teaching cultural competence.

CHANGING DEMOGRAPHICS OF STUDENTS AND HEALTH CARE PROFESSIONALS

The projected increase in immigration, globalization, and minority population growth has the potential to enrich the diversity of the nursing profession and to help meet the needs of an expanding culturally diverse society (Barbee & Gibson, 2001; Bessent, 1997; DHHS, 2000; Griffiths & Tagliareni, 1999; Tucker-Allen & Long, 1999; Villaruel, Canales, & Torres, 2001; Yoder, 2001). What has actually occurred is that the dramatic shift in demographics, the restructured workforce, and a less academically prepared college applicant pool have created a more diverse nursing applicant pool (Kelly, 1997; Tayebi, Moore-Jazayeri, & Maynard, 1998). Nursing students today represent greater diversity in age, ethnicity and race, gender, primary language, prior educational experience, family's educational background, prior work experience, and enrollment status than ever before (Jeffreys, 2004).

Today's student profile characteristics can be examined to predict the potential future impact on the nursing profession (see Table 1.1). For example, recent nursing enrollment trends suggest a steady increase among some minority groups, yet no increase has been noted among Hispanic groups (Antonio, 2001; Heller, Oros, & Durney-Crowley, 2000; Villaruel, Canales, & Torres, 2001). As a result, the number of Hispanic nurses is grossly disproportionate to client populations, demanding urgent and innovative recruitment efforts. Recruitment of diverse, nontraditional student populations does not assure program completion, licensure, or

Table 1.1   Select Nursing Student Trends and Potential Future Impact on the Nursing Profession

Variable	Select nursing student trends	Potential future impact on the nursing profession
Age	Consistent with global and multidisciplinary trends, the enrollment of older students in nursing programs has increased since the mid-1990s with projected increases to persist in the future.	Age at entry into the nursing profession will be older, resulting in decreased number of work years until retirement.
Ethnicity and race	*Enrollment:* Recent nursing enrollment trends suggest a steady increase among some minority groups; however, no increase has been noted among Hispanic groups. *Retention:* Minority groups incur higher attrition rates than nonminority groups.	Currently, white, non-Hispanic nurses of European-American heritage represent approximately 90% of all registered nurses in the United States. Mismatches between the cultural diversity in society and diversity within the nursing profession will persist into the future unless strategies for recruitment and retention are more successful.
Gender	*Men:* Although the numbers of men in nursing are increasing, they remain an underrepresented minority (6%). *Women:* Support for women entering the workforce has shifted away from encouraging traditional female professions.	Men will continue to be disproportionately underrepresented in nursing. Many academically well-qualified male and female high school students with a potential interest in nursing may never enter the nursing profession.
Language	*Enrollment:* Consistent with global and national trends in higher education, nursing programs in the United States and Canada have experienced an increase in English as a second language (ESL) populations since the mid-1990s. *Retention:* ESL student populations have unique learning needs and incur higher attrition rates.	Although individuals with personal lived experiences in other cultures and languages can potentially meet the needs of linguistically diverse and culturally diverse client populations, they will still be disproportionately represented within the nursing profession.

(continued)

Table 1.1 (*Continued*)

Variable	Select nursing student trends	Potential future impact on the nursing profession
Prior educational experience	Consistent with trends in higher education. Worldwide, prior educational experiences are increasingly diverse with an academically less prepared applicant pool. Increases in the number of second-degree individuals have been noted. *Retention:* Academically underprepared students incur higher attrition rates.	Nurses with degrees in other fields can enrich the nursing profession by blending multidisciplinary approaches into nursing. Nurses with academically diverse experiences may broaden the overall perspective, especially with socioeconomic and educationally diverse client populations.
Family's educational background	Nursing programs have also seen an increase in first-generation college students, especially among student groups traditionally underrepresented in nursing. *Retention:* First-generation college students incur higher attrition rates.	First-generation college students who become nurses have the potential to enrich the diversity of the nursing profession and reach out to various socioeconomic and educationally diverse client populations.
Prior work experience	A restructured workforce, welfare-to-work initiatives, displaced homemakers, popularity of midlife career changes, and health care career ladder programs have expanded the nursing applicant pool, increasing its diversity in prior work experience. Many students work full or part time. *Retention:* Work–family–school conflicts may interfere with academic success and retention.	New graduate nurses may enter the nursing profession with various prior work experiences that have the potential to enrich the nursing profession.
Enrollment status	Almost half of all college students attend part time. The number of part-time nursing students, especially those with multiple role responsibilities (work, family), has increased. *Retention:* Work–family–school conflicts may interfere with academic success and retention.	Part-time students will take longer to complete their education. Entry into practice will be delayed, and total number of potential work years in nursing will be decreased.

entry into the professional workforce. In fact, attrition is higher among nontraditional student populations. Therefore, intensive recruitment efforts must be partnered with concentrated efforts aimed at enhancing academic achievement, professional integration, satisfaction, retention, graduation, and entry into the nursing professional workforce.

Unfortunately, current employment trends in nursing indicate high turnover rates with nurses moving from workplace to workplace. High attrition rates for new nurses leaving the nursing profession are also a major concern. The nursing shortage, high acuity of patient care, diminished resources, and an aging society emphasize the need to prioritize retention of nurses in the workplace. Alleviating the nursing shortage, optimizing opportunities for career advancement, offering incentives for educational advancement, and striving to promote professional (and workplace) satisfaction are broad objectives aimed at facilitating nurse retention.

The recruitment of foreign nurses has been one strategy implemented to alleviate the nursing shortage that has contributed to the changing profile characteristics of professional nurses. Foreign nurses are a heterogeneous group, representing much diversity in profile characteristics and in prior work experiences as a registered nurse. The recruitment of foreign nurses must incorporate culturally congruent strategies to ease the transition into the workplace setting, create multicultural workplace harmony, and promote professional satisfaction and opportunities for career advancement. Bridging the gaps between diverse groups of nurses is essential to preventing multicultural workplace conflict and promoting multicultural workplace harmony.

PREPARING CULTURALLY COMPETENT HEALTH CARE PROFESSIONALS

Goals of culturally congruent health care and multicultural workplace harmony can only be achieved by preparing health care professionals to actively engage in the process of cultural competence. Adequate preparation necessitates a diagnostic-prescriptive plan guided by a comprehensive understanding of the teaching–learning process of cultural competency development. Such a comprehensive plan must incorporate a detailed assessment and understanding of learner characteristics. Each learner characteristic provides vital information that is integral to determining special needs and strengths.

Meeting the needs of culturally diverse learners is a growing challenge in academia, the professional workplace, and within professional associations. Because all students, nurses, and other health professionals belong to one or more cultural groups before entering professional education, they bring their patterns of learned values, beliefs, and behaviors into the academic and professional setting. Values are standards that have eminent worth, meaning, and importance in one's life; values guide behavior. These culture values are the "powerful directive forces that give order and meaning to people's thinking, decisions, and actions" (Leininger, 1995a). Culture values guide thinking, decisions, and actions within the student and/or nurse role, as well as other in aspects of their lives. Students, nurses, and other health professionals also hold numerous beliefs (ideas, convictions, philosophical opinions, or tenets) that are accepted as true without requiring evidence or proof. Beliefs are often unconsciously accepted as truths (Purnell & Paulanka, 2003).

CVB unconsciously and consciously guide thinking, decisions, and actions that ultimately affect the process and the outcomes of learning. High levels of cultural congruence serve as a bridge to promoting positive learning experiences and positive academic and/or psychological outcomes; high levels of cultural incongruence are proposed as inversely related to positive learning experiences and academic and/or psychological outcomes (Jeffreys, 2004). Cultural congruence refers to the degree of fit between the learner's values and beliefs and the values and beliefs of their surrounding environment (Constantine, Robinson, Wilton, & Caldwell, 2002; Constantine & Watt, 2002; Gloria & Kurpius, 1996). Here, the surrounding environment refers to the environment of nursing education within the nursing profession and the educational institution, workplace, or professional association setting.

Nursing is a unique culture that reflects its own cultural style. Cultural styles are the "recurring elements, expressions, and qualities that characterize a designated cultural group through their series of action-patterns, beliefs, and values" (Leininger, 1994a, p. 155). The dominant values and norms of a cultural group guide the development of cultural styles (Leininger, 1994a). Currently (within the United States), the culture of nursing reflects many of the dominant societal values and beliefs held in the United States. Similarly, nursing education reflects many of the Western European value system predominant in U.S. universities. Because nursing has its own set of CVB, students must become enculturated into nursing. *Enculturation* is a learning process whereby students learn to take on or live by the values, norms, and expectations of the nursing profession (Leininger, 2002a). Sufficient assistance during enculturation adjustment can minimize acculturation stress and enhance enculturation. Unfortunately, cultural competence as a priority professional value received delayed popularity among the nursing profession overall, with little emphasis or inclusion in nursing curricula, practice, research, theory, administration, and the literature. Consequently, today's nurse educators may be inadequately prepared to enculturate students into the new era of the nursing profession that embraces cultural diversity and supports cultural competence development.

Although increases in culturally diverse students have been noted in higher education and in nursing, the values and beliefs underlying nursing education have been slow to change in accordance with changing student population needs. Ethnocentric tendencies and cultural blindness have been major obstacles to the needed changes in nursing education. Ethnocentric tendencies refer to the belief that the values and beliefs traditionally held within nursing education are supreme. Consequently, traditional teaching–learning practices are upheld. Too often, cultural blindness exists in nursing education. Within the context of nursing education, *cultural blindness* is the inability to recognize the different CVB that exist among diverse student populations. Because cultural blindness does not acknowledge that differences exist, cultural imposition of dominant nursing education values and beliefs undoubtedly occur. Cultural imposition can cause cultural shock, cultural clashes, cultural pain, and cultural assault among students whose CVB are incongruent with the dominant nursing CVB (Jeffreys, 2004).

Nurse educators are challenged to explore various CVB within nursing, nursing education, higher education, and student cultures, and to make culturally sensitive and appropriate decisions, actions, and innovations. Table 1.2 selectively compares and contrasts CVB of nursing education, higher education, and four other cultural groups. Based on a review of the literature, traditional views within the identified cultures were included but are in no way meant to stereotype individuals within the cultures. Readers are cautioned about making stereotypes and are reminded to explore CVB of individual learners. It is beyond the scope of this book to provide in-depth explanations about each category, yet the importance of an in-depth understanding must be recognized. The selective approach is meant to spark interest, stimulate awareness, and encourage further exploration among educators before attempting the design of culturally relevant and congruent educational strategies. This approach is critical because the need to understand, respect, maintain, and support the different CVB of culturally diverse learners is a precursor to culturally relevant and competent education (Abrums & Leppa, 2001; Crow, 1993; Davidhizar, Dowd, & Giger, 1998; Labun, 2002; Manifold & Rambur, 2001; Rew, 1996; Sommer, 2001; Tucker-Allen & Long, 1999; Villaruel, Canales, & Torres, 2001; Weaver, 2001; Williams & Calvillo, 2002; Yoder, 1996; Yoder & Saylor, 2002; Yurkovich, 2001).

The teaching–learning process of cultural competence must consider the various philosophies and approaches to learning. Whether the teacher is perceived to be an authority figure, partner, coach, mentor, professional,

Table 1.2 Comparison of Select Cultural Values and Beliefs

	Nursing Education	Higher Education	Chinese American	African American	Mexican American	Irish American
Orientation	Individual	Individual	Group	Group	Group	Individual
Time Perception	Present and future oriented. Punctuality valued.	Present and future oriented. Punctuality valued.	History of past important. Traditionally, lateness for appointments is expected. More recently, lateness is considered rude.	Present oriented. Punctuality less important.	Present oriented. Relaxed punctuality.	Past, present, future. Flexible sense of time.
Verbal Communication	Direct, specific, and quick communication preferred. Expects individuals to indicate when something is not understood.	Depending on discipline, may have more or less elaboration and speed may not be as much of a priority as in the fast-paced health care setting common to nursing.	Moderate to low tones preferred. Loud tone associated with anger. Answers "yes" when asked if something is understood. Reluctant to talk about feelings and views.	Loud tones (in comparison to other cultures) are preferred. Views and feelings are shared openly with family and trusted friends.	Personal topics may be taboo. Feelings and views only shared with trusted family and friends. "Small talk" expected to begin communication encounter.	Low contextual language where meaning is explicit rather than implicit. Personal topics are private. Thoughts and feelings shared only with close family and friends.
Nonverbal Communication	Most often consistent with dominant societal values, such as direct eye contact, handshaking, and spatial distances.	Most often consistent with dominant societal values, such as direct eye contact, handshaking, and spatial distances.	Avoid direct eye contact, especially with persons of authority and highly respected individuals.	Direct eye contact is sometimes perceived as aggressive.	Avoid direct eye contact, especially with persons of authority and highly respected individuals. Handshaking demonstrates respect.	Direct eye contact is maintained, indicating respect and trust.

(continued)

Household Responsibilities	The "traditional" student did not have household or outside responsibilities. Student role is primary.	The "traditional" student did not have household or outside responsibilities. Student role is primary. Community colleges have expanded services available to accommodate adult learner with multiple role responsibilities. Examples: weekend or evening college, day care center.	Household responsibilities shared; however, specific roles expected based on gender. Male is head of family.	Household responsibilities may be divided among men, women, and children. Woman is often head of family.	Household responsibilities mainly part of female role. Male dominance with male as head of family. Modesty.
Health	Professes "holistic" view of health but still strongly based on medical model with focus on symptom alleviation, use of technology, and Western medicine.	Health is not the major focus of institutions of higher education. In recent years, many colleges have eliminated or relaxed graduation requirements for courses in health, fitness, and/or physical education.	Balance between "yin and yang."	"Health is viewed as a harmony with nature."	Balance between "hot and cold."
Nurse	"Professional." Seeking more respect from other health professionals and society.	In comparison to other disciplines, nursing had a late start in higher education. May be viewed as a vocation rather than profession.	Respected as authority figures after physicians. Nurses with advanced education are more highly respected than are nurses with less education.	Respected member of the health care team but less important than physicians.	Respected member of the health care team; however, often viewed as an outsider.

Additional column (rightmost):

Household Responsibilities	Traditionally, household responsibilities part of female role; however, in recent years, responsibilities shared between men and women.
Health	Determined by external forces.
Nurse	Nurses are respected as members of a service-oriented field or "occupation."

17

Table 1.2 *(Continued)*

	Nursing Education	Higher Education	Chinese American	African American	Mexican American	Irish American
Education	Within the nursing culture, disputes surrounding minimal educational requirements still persist.	Minimal education for tenure and promotion is the doctorate, although master's degree may be minimal at the community colleges.	Highly valued, especially a college education.	Highly valued, especially a college education	Education is valued; however, access to college education has been limited historically. Families often expect females to put family first.	Education is highly valued.
Teaching and Learning	Traditional pedagogy viewed teacher as "authority" who "transmits" learning to student. Newer proponents of andragogy view teacher as partner or facilitator of learning who implements learner-centered approaches.	Traditional pedagogy viewed teacher as "authority" who "transmits" learning to student. Newer proponents of andragogy view teacher as partner or facilitator of learning who implements learner-centered approaches. Teaching role and load has greater emphasis at community colleges. Teaching role may be secondary to scholarly activity, publication, and research at senior colleges and research institutions.	Authority figure. True equality does not exist; therefore, concept of "partner" in learning may be difficult to comprehend. High expectation within group to excel academically.	Respected authority figure. Historically, unequal opportunities for advancing education Disproportionate numbers receive primary and secondary education in at-risk school districts (educational disadvantaged).	Teacher is viewed as a highly respected superior. Rote learning and memorization predominates education in Mexico, with little emphasis on practical application, analysis, and synthesis.	Respected professional.
Work Habits	Speed, accuracy, quality, and cost effectiveness are valued. Completion of tasks and "keeping busy" traditionally valued.	"Keeping busy" is less valued than high-quality, scholarly productivity, especially at senior colleges and research institutions.	Speed in working is not a priority. Hard work is valued.	Hard work is valued.	Work is secondary to family and other life activities. May be uncomfortable with authority persons checking work.	Hard work highly valued.

18

Autonomy	Competition with authority. Assertive. Autonomous decision making within the scope of nursing practice expected.	Competitive, assertive. Academic freedom highly valued. Democratic governance, faculty-developed curricula, and professional unions/organizations valued.	Defers to person in authority, often seeking approval before making decisions. Avoids conflict and values harmony.	Self-reliance and autonomy encouraged within group. Past discrimination experiences may discourage autonomy. Females are often heads of household and decision makers.	Defers to person in authority with males as dominant decision makers. Input of others is considered in decision making. Autonomy for females is more difficult than for males. Avoids competition and conflict.	Autonomy and independence outside the family is encouraged, while family loyalty is still maintained.
Help-Seeking Behaviors	Individual is expected to initiate help-seeking behaviors.	Individual is expected to initiate help-seeking behaviors.	Stigma for seeking help for emotional disorders and stress. May be reluctant to approach for help by attempting to "save face."	Varied. May seek help within own social network before seeking outside help.	Varied. May seek help within own social network before seeking outside help.	May delay seeking help. Denial of problems is a way of coping with physical and emotional problems.
Persistence	Nursing is "hard work." Withdrawal from a nursing course is acceptable for academic and/or personal circumstances and should be decided by the individual.	Among disciplines outside of nursing, nursing may not be perceived as "hard work" or academically rigorous/challenging work for academically strong students. Views on withdrawal similar to nursing education.	Hard work is highly respected. Withdrawal decisions may be difficult and may include the family.	Withdrawal decisions may be difficult, especially if families have sacrificed greatly to assist student with educational endeavors.	Withdrawal decisions may be difficult, especially if families have sacrificed greatly to assist student with educational endeavors. Decisions may include the family. Withdrawal would be acceptable if interfering with family responsibilities.	Withdrawal decisions may be difficult because academic or personal problem must first be acknowledged.

Information from Andrews & Boyle, 1999; Campinha-Bacote, 1998; Leininger & McFarland, 2002; Purnell & Paulanka, 2003. Adapted from Jeffreys, M.R. (2004). *Nursing student retention: Understanding the process & making a difference.* New York, Springer. Used by permission, Springer Publishing Company, Inc., 10036.

or member of a service occupation will influence the teaching–learning process (see Table 1.2). Preferred teaching–learning styles may be active (learner centered) or passive (teacher centered). Teaching–learning strategies perceived as fun and likable by some may be perceived as aggressive (debate), competitive (gaming), threatening (web-based, role-playing, or small-group activity), boring (rote memorization), and/or irrelevant by others. Learner goals and philosophies that emphasize the "process" of learning focus on the journey of "becoming" cultural competent through the integration of cognitive, practical, and affective learning. Process learners recognize that the journey itself is the "learning"; obstacles, mistakes, and hardships along the way are part of the expected developmental process that requires extra effort, sincere commitment, motivation, and persistence. Process learners realize that there is no final end product labeled "cultural competence," rather cultural competence is dynamic and ongoing. In contrast, "product" learners are focused on obtaining an end product through the mastery of content. Memorizing a multitude of "facts" about a culture becomes important rather than comprehensively understanding, applying, and appreciating the cultural context or rationale behind the "fact." There is a lack of concern with how to learn to apply knowledge and develop skills, and even less concern with affective learning (values, attitudes, and beliefs). Product learners would be greatly disturbed, dissatisfied, and poorly motivated with an approach that views the end point for becoming culturally competent as infinite.

Perceived barriers to learning, mismatches in teacher–learner expectations, and poor learning experiences will hinder the learning process of cultural competence. For example, faculty beliefs that nonminority students are less confident in caring for culturally different clients than minority students are stereotypical and inaccurate (Jeffreys, 2000; Jeffreys & Smodlaka, 1998, 1999a, 1999b; Lim, Downie, & Nathan, 2004). Similarly, the belief that minority nurses are intrinsically equipped to care for culturally diverse clients is also inaccurate, negating the uniqueness of the many cultures that comprise the federally recognized "minority" group categories and disregarding the many cultures that comprise nonminority groups. The danger is that minority students' and nurses' special needs concerning learning to provide culturally congruent care for many different groups of culturally different clients (different in culture from care provider) may be ignored. Expectations that are more, less, or different based solely on ethnic or racial background are grossly inadequate because other diverse profile characteristics and their potential influence on learning must be objectively appraised.

Meeting the needs of learners representing diversity in age, ethnicity and race, gender, primary language, prior educational experience, family's educational background, prior work experience, and/or enrollment means embracing a broader, inclusive worldview that appreciates various forms of diversity. Awareness of how each profile variable can potentially influence learning is a necessary first step in understanding the multidimensional process of cultural competence education. For example, the learning needs and expectations of foreign-educated learners may be quite different from what educators initially perceive, creating an obstacle for learning, achievement, and satisfaction (Jalili-Grenier & Chase, 1997). Acculturation stress, adaptation, assimilation, CVB toward education, experiences with second language, and expectations can greatly impact learning and achievement (Flege & Liu, 2001; Fuertes & Westbrook, 1996; Jalili-Grenier & Chase, 1997; Kataoka-Yahiro & Abriam-Yago, 1997; Kurz, 1993; Manifold & Rambur, 2001; Olenchak & Hebert, 2002; Smart & Smart, 1995; Upton & Lee-Thompson, 2001). Other stressors that may affect specific subgroups in nursing include perceived cultural incongruence (Constantine, Robinson, Wilton, & Caldwell, 2002; Maville & Huerta, 1997); perceived (or fear of) discrimination and bias (Kirkland, 1998); student (learner) role incongruence (Chartrand, 1990); maternal role stress (Gigliotti, 1999, 2001); perceived multiple role stress (Courage & Godbey, 1992; Gigliotti, 1999, 2001; Greenhaus & Beutell, 1985; Lambert & Nugent, 1994; Loerch, Russell, & Rush, 1989); and gender role identity stress (Baker, 2001; Constantine & Watt, 2002; Patterson & Morin, 2002; Streubert, 1994). In addition, students who work in the health care field as unlicensed personnel, licensed practical nurses (LPNs), or health care paraprofessionals may have difficulty adjusting to a new role, new worldview, and critical thinking and decision making within a nursing perspective that is guided by the professional scope of nursing practice. New graduate nurses may experience reality shock with their new professional role, workload, and responsibilities; experienced nurses may encounter burnout.

CULTURAL COMPETENCE AND CONFIDENCE

Despite the numerous complexities, changes, and challenges faced by many nursing students and nurses today, some individuals are more actively engaged in cultural competence development, whereas others are not. Some individuals are more motivated to pursue cultural competence development and are more committed to the goal of culturally congruent care than others. Therefore, the evaluation of factors that may influence motivation, persistence, and commitment for cultural competency development is a necessary precursor to any educational design strategy. Confidence (self-efficacy) is one such factor that is emphasized in this book. According to Bandura (1986), the construct of self-efficacy is the individuals' perceived confidence for learning or performing specific tasks or skills necessary to achieve a particular goal. Furthermore, self-efficacy is the belief that one can perform or succeed at learning a specific task, despite obstacles and hardships, and will expend whatever energy is necessary to accomplish the task (Bandura, 1986). Consequently, confidence is inextricably linked as a major component in cultural competence development and an influencing factor in the achievement of culturally congruent care. Chapter 2 proposes a new conceptual model to understand and guide cultural competence education, research, and practice.

KEY POINT SUMMARY

- Rapid growth in worldwide migration, changes in demographic patterns, varying fertility rates, increased numbers of multiracial and multiethnic individuals, and advanced technology contribute to cultural evolution.
- Cultural evolution refers to the process of cultural growth and change within a society.
- Culturally congruent health care refers to health care that is customized to fit with the client's cultural values, beliefs, traditions, practices, and lifestyle.
- Cultural competence is a multidimensional process that aims to achieve culturally congruent health care.
- Professional goals, societal needs, ethical considerations, and legal issues all declare the need to prioritize cultural competence development, necessitating a conscious, committed, and transformational change in current nursing practice, education, and research.
- Two major barriers prevent a rapid effective transformation through transcultural education: (a) lack of faculty and advanced practice nurses formally prepared in transcultural nursing and in the teaching of transcultural nursing, and (b) limited research evaluating the effectiveness of teaching interventions on the development of cultural competence.
- Changing demographics of students and health care professionals, as well as the severe shortage of nurses and nursing faculty, further complicate effective transformation.
- Goals of culturally congruent health care and multicultural workplace harmony can only be achieved by preparing (teaching) health care professionals to actively engage in the (learning) process of cultural competence.

- Meeting the needs of learners representing diversity in age, ethnicity and race, gender, primary language, prior educational experience, family's educational background, prior work experience, and/or enrollment means embracing a broader, inclusive worldview that appreciates various forms of diversity and must consider the various philosophies and approaches to learning.
- Despite the numerous complexities, changes, and challenges faced by many nursing students and nurses today, some individuals are more motivated and actively engaged in cultural competence development, whereas others are not.
- Confidence (self-efficacy) is an important factor that may influence motivation, persistence, and commitment for cultural competency development.

A Model to Guide Cultural Competence Education

Providing culturally specific and congruent care to the myriad culturally diverse populations is a growing professional challenge. The expanding number of immigrant populations seeking health care, compounded by the growing diverse nursing student population, predicted in the future suggests that increasingly professional nurses will care for clients who are "culturally different." *Culturally different* clients are clients whose racial, ethnic, gender, socioeconomic, and/or religious backgrounds and/or identities are different from the health care professional or student. For educators, preparing culturally diverse nursing students to care competently for culturally different clients will be even more challenging. For health care professionals and health care institutions (HCIs), the challenge is to provide educational opportunities to enhance the cultural competency of health care professionals so that quality outcome indicators such as enhanced client satisfaction and positive health outcomes may be achieved.

Although the need to prepare students and health professionals to become culturally sensitive and competent is extremely urgent, research in the area of understanding the teaching–learning process of cultural competency has been limited. Research priorities, guided by conceptual models must shift toward strategies aimed at maximizing learner strengths, identifying learner weaknesses, and developing diagnostic-prescriptive teaching interventions. A conceptual model that depicts the multidimensional components of the teaching–learning process of cultural competency could serve as a valuable cognitive map to guide educators, researchers, and learners. Furthermore, a model that addresses factors that influence learning, motivation, persistence, and commitment for cultural competency development would offer a more comprehensive approach.

Such an approach must recognize that despite the learning opportunities presented to students, nurses, and other health professionals, some individuals persist at cultural competency development, whereas others do not. According to Bandura (1986), learning and motivation for learning are directly influenced by self-efficacy perceptions (confidence). *Self-efficacy* is the perceived confidence for learning or performing specific tasks or skills necessary to achieve a particular goal. Moreover, self-efficacy is the belief that one can perform or succeed at learning a specific task, despite obstacles and hardships, and will expend whatever energy is necessary to accomplish the task (Bandura, 1986). Self-efficacy has been strongly linked to persistence behaviors and motivation. *Motivation* has been described as "the 'power within' that will generate actions that will result in his or her success" (Stage & Hossler, 2000, p. 173). Motivation to engage in the process of becoming culturally competent has been termed *cultural desire*; cultural desire has been viewed as the "pivotal construct of cultural competence" (Campinha-Bacote, 2003, p. 14). As a determinant of performance, persistence, motivation, and the self-regulation of learning, self-efficacy (perceived confidence) is a major component in learning (Bandura, 1982, 1986, 1995, 1996, 1997; Maddux, 1995; Multon, Brown, & Lent, 1991; Pintrich & Garcia, 1994; Zimmerman, 1996). Consequently, confidence is a vital component in the process of learning cultural competence (Box 2.1).

The Cultural Competence and Confidence (CCC) model (see Figure 2.1) aims to interrelate concepts that explain, describe, influence, and/or predict the phenomenon of learning (developing) cultural competence and incorporates the construct of transcultural self-efficacy (confidence) as a major influencing factor. *Transcultural self-efficacy* (TSE) is the perceived confidence for performing or learning general transcultural nursing skills among culturally different clients. *Cultural competence* is defined as a multidimensional learning process that integrates transcultural skills in all three dimensions (cognitive, practical, and affective), involves TSE (confidence) as a major influencing factor, and aims to achieve culturally congruent care. The term *learning process* emphasizes that the cognitive, practical, and affective dimensions of TSE and transcultural skill development can change over time as a result of formalized education and other learning experiences.

The CCC model is proposed to provide an organizing framework for understanding the multidimensional process of cultural competence development by succinctly illustrating major components of the learning process (see Figure 2.1). This chapter begins by describing the initial conceptualization surrounding model development. Key terms and underlying assumptions are introduced. A close-up view of TSE, cultural

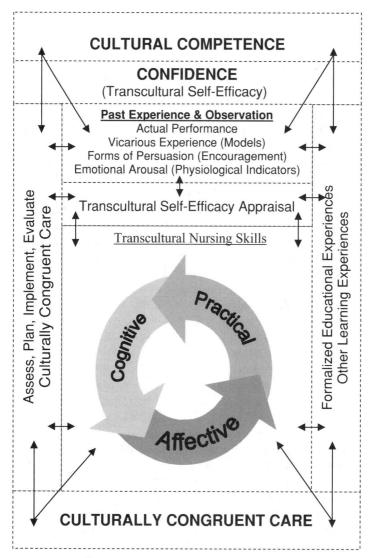

Figure 2.1 Jeffreys' Cultural Competence and Confidence (CCC) model.

competence, and culturally congruent care is depicted through the TSE Pathway (see Figure 2.2), thereby expanding on the major components of the CCC model. An overview of the conceptual model and essential background information concludes the chapter. Lastly, the model is brought to life through a realistic "Educator-in-Action" vignette featuring

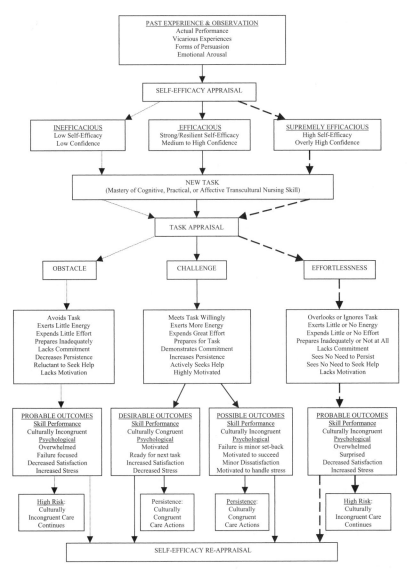

Figure 2.2 Transcultural Self-Efficacy (TSE) Pathway. Adapted from Jeffreys, M. R. (2004). *Nursing student retention: Understanding the process and making a difference.* New York, Springer. Used by permission, Springer Publishing Company, Inc., NY 10036.

cultural competence education in the health care institution (hospital setting).

BEGINNING ROOTS, OBSERVATIONS, AND INITIAL CONCEPTUALIZATION

A brief discussion of the CCC model's beginning roots from the author's observations, initial ideas, conceptualization, empirical support, and changes over time aims to demonstrate that the CCC model is developmental, tentative, dynamic, and continually evolving as new data become available. The model presents one perspective that will hopefully spark further inquiry into the complex yet extremely important process of developing cultural competence.

Initial ideas often evolve from multiple sources. An area of interest may be based on formal or informal observations or derived from issues in professional nursing. In the present case, both informal and formal observations led to the author's design of a series of studies and the development of the CCC model. Early, informal observations noted that confidence, lack of confidence, or overconfidence was an intriguingly complex phenomenon that could influence learning and performance. This observation was especially noted in interactions with aquaphobics and athletes, prior to becoming a registered nurse. Despite cognitive knowledge and psychomotor ability, learning and performance were often influenced by confidence level either directly or indirectly. Direct effects were manifested through performance outcomes; indirect effects included varying levels of avoidance behaviors, persistence, indifference, commitment, effort, satisfaction, fear, and/or stress.

Later, as an undergraduate nursing student, the author also informally observed confidence to be a factor in learning, performance, and overall success. Fellow nursing students who lacked confidence often performed poorly, despite his or her knowledge, critical thinking ability, manual dexterity, and speaking ability. Others became frustrated, simply gave up trying, and dropped out. Positive-thinking peers who studied and practiced skills seemed to like nursing more and achieve better outcomes. When working as a staff nurse, the author also noted confidence to be a factor influencing professional nursing practice, career satisfaction, and career advancement. Among clients, confidence levels were also seen as variables influencing client outcomes. These observations were informal, yet impressionable.

Subsequent observations as a nursing faculty member found confidence to be an important component in nursing student achievement, persistence, retention, and success. Interest in enhancing nursing student achievement, persistence, retention, and success became a focused area of inquiry. Review of the literature in education and psychology revealed Bandura's (1986) social cognitive theory; an underlying component of social cognitive theory was self-efficacy (the perceived confidence for learning or performing specific tasks or skills necessary to achieve a particular goal). Self-efficacy is task or domain specific, and has been correlated with academic achievement, persistence, retention, and success; hence, self-efficacy became a targeted variable for the author's study within the context of nursing education.

During the author's doctoral dissertation study concerning first-semester nontraditional associate degree student achievement and retention, individual item review of perceived self-efficacy for 60 select nursing skills suggested that students were least confident about learning specific communications skills than they were about skills in other categories (Jeffreys, 1993). Eight of the 10 communication items received responses ranking in the 30th percentile (least confident). More specifically, overall less confidence was reported for interviewing a client about "financial concerns," "religious practices and beliefs," and "ethnic food preferences." These were the only items that dealt with cultural issues such as socioeconomic status (class), religion, and ethnicity.

Why were students least confident about communication? Why were students less confident about items related to cultural issues? How would students have responded to items that further delineated the various dimensions of culture? According to Bandura (1986), individuals with low confidence are at greater risk for task avoidance and decreased commitment. If students are avoiding tasks or less committed to tasks associated with culture, then how can cultural assessments, cultural-specific nursing care, culturally congruent care, and cultural competence be achieved? Furthermore, cultural assessments must begin with effective transcultural communication. Effective transcultural communication necessitates awareness, sensitivity, knowledge, and skills. "Transcultural" implies bridging of significant differences in cultural communication styles, beliefs, or practices (Kavanagh & Kennedy, 1992). If students are less confident about general communication skills, how will cultural assessments be performed (or will they be performed)? The obvious gaps and lowered confidence raised the important question "What teaching interventions are needed to promote culturally congruent care?"

Interest in learning more about students' self-efficacy perceptions concerning specific transcultural nursing skills necessary for developing cultural competence became the author's new focused domain of inquiry. Specifically, the area of interest was to develop a composite of students' needs, values, attitudes, and skills related to transcultural nursing care and the assessment of their changes (outcomes) over time. Assessing students' needs, strengths, weaknesses, and perceptions would be the necessary precursor to the design of any teaching interventions. "Effective teaching and learning is further enhanced by frequent and ongoing evaluations of students and by adapting educational instruction based on outcome assessments" (Jeffreys & Smodlaka, 1996, p. 47). The author believed that the initial and ongoing assessment of students' self-efficacy perceptions (confidence) concerning culture care of diverse individuals would be a valuable component in transcultural nursing education. Subsequently, several studies were undertaken to explore, measure, and evaluate learners' TSE perceptions (Jeffreys, 2000; Jeffreys & Smodlaka, 1996, 1998, 1999a, 1999b). (Chapter 3 discusses measuring and evaluating learners through the use of the Transcultural Self-Efficacy Tool.) A description of the CCC model is presented in the following sections.

KEY TERMS

To develop a common knowledge base and avoid discrepancies in definitions, Table 2.1 defines key terms important in understanding the CCC model.

PURPOSE AND GOAL OF THE MODEL

The CCC model presents an organizing framework for examining the multidimensional factors involved in the process of learning cultural competence in order to identify at-risk individuals, develop diagnostic-prescriptive strategies to facilitate learning, guide innovations in teaching and educational research, and evaluate strategy effectiveness. The main goal of the model is to promote culturally congruent care through the development of cultural competence. Cultural competence is influenced by TSE; the learning of transcultural nursing skills (cognitive, practical, and affective), formalized educational experiences, and other learning experiences. Although several models have been proposed to describe the process of cultural competence (Campinha-Bacote, 2003; Purnell, 2003) or the process of achieving culturally congruent care through the assessment of cultural diversity and universality (Leininger, 2002a, 2002c), the CCC model focuses specifically on learning as influenced by TSE. Hence, TSE is proposed as a new construct vital to the process of cultural competence and culturally congruent care. The model is tentative and will require modification when new data become available.

Table 2.1   Key Terms Associated With the Cultural Competence
and Confidence (CCC) Model

Transcultural self-efficacy is the perceived confidence for performing or learning transcultural nursing skills. It is the degree to which individuals perceive they have the ability to perform the specific transcultural nursing skills needed for culturally competent and congruent care (Jeffreys, 2000).

Transcultural nursing skills are those skills necessary for assessing, planning, implementing, and evaluating culturally congruent care. Transcultural nursing skills include cognitive, practical, and affective dimensions (Jeffreys, 2000).

Culturally congruent care is health care that is customized to fit with the client's cultural values, beliefs, traditions, practices, and lifestyle. Clients may include individuals, families, groups, institutions, and organizations. According to Leininger (1991a), **culturally congruent nursing care** refers to "those cognitively based assistive, supportive, facilitative, or enabling acts or decisions that are tailor-made to fit with an individual's, group's, or institution's cultural values, beliefs, and lifeways in order to provide meaningful, beneficial, and satisfying health care, or well-being services" (p. 49).

Cultural competence is a multidimensional learning process that integrates transcultural skills in all three dimensions (cognitive, practical, and affective), involves transcultural self-efficacy (confidence) as a major influencing factor, and aims to achieve culturally congruent care. **Cultural competence in nursing** is a multidimensional learning process that integrates transcultural nursing skills in all three dimensions (cognitive, practical, and affective), involves transcultural self-efficacy (confidence), and aims to achieve culturally congruent nursing care. The term **learning process** emphasizes that the cognitive, practical, and affective dimensions of transcultural self-efficacy can change over time as a result of formalized education and other learning experiences.

The **cognitive learning dimension** is a learning dimension that focuses on knowledge outcomes, intellectual abilities, and skills. Within the context of transcultural learning, cognitive learning skills include knowledge and comprehension about ways in which cultural factors may influence professional nursing care among clients of different cultural backgrounds and throughout various phases of the life cycle. The term **different cultural backgrounds** refers to clients representing various different racial, ethnic, gender, socioeconomic, and religious groups.

The **practical learning dimension** is similar to the psychomotor learning domain and focuses on motor skills or practical application of skills. Within the context of transcultural learning, practical learning skills refer to communication skills (verbal and nonverbal) needed to interview clients of different cultural backgrounds about their values and beliefs.

The **affective learning dimension** is a learning dimension concerned with attitudes, values, and beliefs, and is considered to be the most important in developing professional values and attitudes. Affective learning includes self-awareness, awareness of cultural gap (differences), acceptance, appreciation, recognition, and advocacy.

ASSUMPTIONS

Based on a review of the literature and previous studies of self-efficacy (Jeffreys, 2000), several assumptions underlie the CCC model:

- Cultural competence is an ongoing, multidimensional learning process that integrates transcultural skills in all three dimensions (cognitive, practical, and affective), involves TSE (confidence) as a major influencing factor, and aims to achieve culturally congruent care.
- TSE is a dynamic construct that changes over time and is influenced by formalized exposure to culture care concepts (transcultural nursing).
- The learning of transcultural nursing skills is influenced by self-efficacy perceptions (confidence).
- The performance of transcultural nursing skill competencies is directly influenced by the adequate learning of such skills and by TSE perceptions.
- The performance of culturally congruent nursing skills is influenced by self-efficacy perceptions and by formalized educational exposure to transcultural nursing care concepts and skills throughout the educational experience.
- All students and nurses (regardless of age, ethnicity, gender, sexual orientation, lifestyle, religion, socioeconomic status, geographic location, or race) require formalized educational experiences to meet culture care needs of diverse individuals.
- The most comprehensive learning involves the integration of cognitive, practical, and affective dimensions.
- Learning in the cognitive, practical, and affective dimensions is paradoxically distinct yet interrelated.
- Learners are most confident about their attitudes (affective dimension) and least confident about their transcultural nursing knowledge (cognitive dimension).
- Novice learners will have lower self-efficacy perceptions than advanced learners.
- Inefficacious individuals are at risk for decreased motivation, lack of commitment, and/or avoidance of cultural considerations when planning and implementing nursing care.
- Supremely efficacious (overly confident) individuals are at risk for inadequate preparation in learning the transcultural nursing skills necessary to provide culturally congruent care.
- Early intervention with at-risk individuals will better prepare nurses to meet cultural competency.

- The greatest change in TSE perceptions will be detected in individuals with low self-efficacy (low confidence) initially, who have then been exposed to formalized transcultural nursing concepts and experiences.

OVERVIEW OF THE CULTURAL COMPETENCE AND CONFIDENCE MODEL

Cultural competence in nursing is a multidimensional learning process that integrates transcultural nursing skills in all three dimensions (cognitive, practical, and affective), involves TSE (confidence), and aims to achieve culturally congruent care. Cognitive, practical, and affective dimensions of TSE can change over time as a result of formalized education and other learning experiences. Each learning dimension is comprised of several underlying factors or concepts. Figure 2.2 traces the proposed influences of TSE on a learner's actions, performance, and persistence for learning tasks associated with cultural competency development and culturally congruent care. TSE appraisal is a key beginning step in this process.

Self-efficacy appraisal is an individualized process influenced by four information sources: actual performances, vicarious experiences, forms of persuasion, and emotional arousal (physiological indices). Actual performances are the strongest source of efficacy information (Bandura, 1986). Successful performances can raise efficacy while unsuccessful performances lower it. Lowered self-efficacy can be psychologically stressful and dissatisfying to nursing students, nurses, and other health care professionals, further negatively impacting motivation, persistence, and cultural competency development. Individuals with low self-efficacy can initially be devastated by failure or poor performance, and further lowered self-efficacy can cause avoidance behaviors (Bandura, 1986, 1997).

Undoubtedly, avoidance behaviors raise numerous professional, ethical, and legal issues; however, the most severe consequence is that avoidance behavior can be dangerous. For example, a student or nurse with low self-efficacy for interviewing a culturally different client about religious and ethnic values, beliefs, and practices concerning food and nutrition may avoid asking important questions. Without adequate cultural assessment, culturally incongruent care can result, causing adverse physical and emotional outcomes to the client. A nurse who reluctantly attempts to interview a culturally different client, avoids cultural-specific assessments, and misinterprets client's statements and actions may fail to recognize the client's cultural pain (Jeffreys, 2005b). Cultural pain refers to the "suffering, discomfort, or being greatly offended by an individual or group who shows a great lack of sensitivity toward another's cultural experience" (Leininger, 2002a, p. 52). In addition to the negative emotional client outcomes, adverse physical client outcomes may occur. If a diabetic client disregards the nurse's suggested diet plan menu because of food taboos, ethnic food preferences, and/or economic constraints, the possible adverse physical health outcomes are numerous. In failing to realize why the client is not adhering to diet recommendations, an inefficacious nurse may be fearful of attempting follow-up diet teaching, lack motivation, avoid help-seeking behaviors, and become increasingly dissatisfied and anxious.

Individuals with strong (realistic) levels of self-efficacy will not be adversely affected by an occasional failure. Such individuals view an occasional failure as a temporary setback or challenge to be overcome with more effort expenditure (Bandura, 1986, 1997). In the previous case example, the realistically strong efficacious student would be motivated to seek extra assistance in the skills lab or request additional supervised opportunities in the clinical setting to ask cultural-specific questions, select culturally appropriate communication style, and seek appropriate resources for culturally congruent food choices. Most likely, such a student (or nurse) would initially take the task seriously, view it with some uncertainty, and exert preparatory efforts before attempting to interview a culturally different client in the clinical setting. Preparatory efforts may include collaboration with health professionals, members of the cultural community, family, and/or client to determine the "best" culturally congruent approach.

In contrast, the supremely efficacious individual (unrealistic in self-appraisal) would view the task without uncertainty, prepare inadequately (or not at all), and potentially jeopardize patient safety if inaccurate assessments are made and appropriate assistance is not sought. Again, unsuccessful performance will lower self-efficacy; however, for the supremely efficacious individual, the goal would be that the task would now be viewed seriously and as a challenge that required adequate preparatory efforts.

Vicarious experience, or modeling, is less influential than actual performance. Models that display effort and perform tasks successfully will be more influential than models completing the task effortlessly. Self-efficacy perceptions will be further enhanced if models are similar to the individual in background and ability (Bandura, 1986; Schunk, 1987). It would be expected that novices (beginning students and new graduate nurses) have less astute skills for observing models. Because beginning students have little or no experience in the domain of nursing, such students will be at risk for selective observations that are myopic, slightly skewed, severely distorted, or limited, thereby increasing the risk for unrealistic self-appraisals. New graduates may be overwhelmed by technical tasks, fast-paced expectations to care for many acutely ill patients, the severe nursing shortage, and lack of sufficient resources. Experienced nurses or other health professionals who are novices in developing cultural competence may also need guidance in observation skills. Through the use of various structured mentoring strategies, more experienced nurses (expert nurses) and educators can enhance the power of modeling on self-efficacy appraisal and development. (Refer to part II of this book for strategies.) By assisting students and novice nurses to develop keen observation skills, educators can have a powerful influence on efficacy appraisal.

Forms of persuasion include positive verbal feedback from peers, teachers, supervisors, mentors, and significant others. Positive persuasion will only enhance efficacy if the individual's subsequent efforts turn out positively (Schunk, 1987). Therefore, positive verbal feedback should be given judiciously and honestly if it is to have any positive impact. In the TSE Pathway (see Figure 2.2), "forms of persuasion" refers to "encouragement by peers, faculty, supervisors, colleagues, mentors, or friends." Encouragement must be realistic, thus incorporating this important dimension of self-efficacy appraisal.

Physiological indices such as elevated pulse rate and sweating may indicate emotional arousal such as anxiety and/or fear. Conscious awareness of anxiety symptoms over a particular task may lower efficacy beliefs (Bandura, 1986, 1997; Schunk, 1987). For example, if a nurse repeatedly experiences anxiety symptoms such as elevated pulse rate and sweating before caring for culturally different clients (despite his or her cognitive and psychomotor ability to perform tasks), then the nurse's efficacy beliefs may be lowered, adversely affecting learning, performance, persistence, motivation, and cultural competency development. Mild anxiety associated with some uncertainty has some benefits in that individuals are more attentive to detail, recognize the need for preparatory actions, and actively seek assistance. Lack of physiological changes would accompany the expected profile of supremely efficacious individuals and adversely affect task performance.

Self-efficacy changes over time in response to new experiences and observations (Bandura, 1989; Gist & Mitchell, 1992; Saks, 1995). Cultural competence development is enhanced through carefully orchestrated education interventions, strategies to increase cultural awareness and desire, opportunities for interaction with culturally different clients, and collaboration with transcultural experts (Campinha-Bacote, 2003; Leininger, 2002a, 2002b; Purnell, 2003). Within the CCC model, formalized educational experiences and client learning experiences that (a) carefully weave cognitive, practical, and affective transcultural nursing skills; (b) encompass assessment, planning, implementation, and evaluation; and

(c) integrate self-efficacy appraisals and diagnostic-specific interventions are essential in cultural competence development and culturally congruent care. Several studies supported that culturally diverse nursing students' self-efficacy perceptions were significantly influenced by their educational and health care experiences. For example, students' course level was statistically significant in influencing perceptions in these studies, which examined changes in TSE perceptions (Jeffreys & Smodlaka, 1996, 1998, 1999a, 1999b; Lim et al., 2004). Novice (beginning) students had overall lower self-efficacy perceptions, whereas advanced (more experienced) students had overall higher self-efficacy perceptions. Ethnic/racial group identity was statistically insignificant, suggesting that self-efficacy measures can be designed to capture the effect of educational experiences across culturally diverse groups; however, further empirical investigation is recommended. Bandura (1995, 1996a) pointed out that the construct of self-efficacy is of vital importance across cultures and should not be confused with Western individualism. Within hospitals and clinical agencies, changes in nurses' TSE perceptions following cultural competence educational interventions have also been reported (Dolgan, 2001; Platter, 2005; Velez, 2005).

Carefully designed self-efficacy measures (survey tools) can be used to appraise the initial self-efficacy levels for particular tasks and skills prior to designing educational interventions. Review of survey data to identify inefficacious and supremely efficacious individuals will allow for early intervention and assistance in enhancing realistic self-efficacy appraisal. Because Bandura (1982, 1989, 1996a, 1996b) recommended situation- or task-specific tools to measure self-efficacy and proposed other guidelines in self-efficacy tool development, educators and researchers should selectively choose a reliable and valid self-efficacy tool specifically matching their research needs. Often, this means that a new tool must be developed. The instrument design process is complex and time consuming; however, specific steps should be followed to enhance the validity and reliability of findings (Jeffreys & Smodlaka, 1996; Waltz, Strickland, & Lenz, 2005). Chapter 3 comprehensively describes an empirically tested tool, the Transcultural Self-Efficacy Tool (TSET), for measurement and evaluation.

KEY POINT SUMMARY

- The CCC model is proposed as an organizing framework for examining the multidimensional factors involved in the process of learning cultural competence in order to identify at-risk individuals, develop diagnostic-prescriptive strategies to facilitate learning, guide innovations in teaching and educational research, and evaluate strategy effectiveness.

- The CCC model interrelates concepts that explain, describe, influence, and/or predict the phenomenon of learning (developing) cultural competence and incorporates the construct of TSE (confidence) as a major influencing factor.

- Cultural competence is a multidimensional learning process that integrates transcultural skills in all three dimensions (cognitive, practical, and affective), involves TSE (confidence) as a major influencing factor, and aims to achieve culturally congruent care.

- Cultural competence is influenced by TSE, the learning of transcultural nursing skills (cognitive, practical, and affective), formalized educational experiences, and other learning experiences.

- Within the CCC model, formalized educational experiences and client learning experiences that (a) carefully weave cognitive, practical, and affective transcultural nursing skills; (b) encompass assessment, planning, implementation, and evaluation; and (c) integrate self-efficacy appraisals and diagnostic-specific interventions are considered essential in cultural competence development and culturally congruent care.

- TSE is the perceived confidence for performing or learning transcultural nursing skills. It is the degree to which individuals perceive they have the ability to perform the specific transcultural nursing skills needed for culturally competent and congruent care.

- The TSE Pathway traces the proposed influences of TSE on a learner's actions, performance, and persistence for learning tasks associated with cultural competency development and culturally congruent care. TSE appraisal is a key beginning step in this process.

- Self-efficacy appraisal is an individualized process influenced by four information sources: actual performances, vicarious experiences, forms of persuasion, and emotional arousal (physiological indices).

- Informal and formal observations, literature reviews, and empirical studies led to the conceptualization surrounding CCC model development.

Box 2.1 Educator-in-Action Vignette

Jeannette, a clinical nurse educator at a hospital, is puzzled by some of the comments written on the anonymous evaluation forms following a hospital-sponsored cultural competence development workshop. Jeannette tells Trudy, another clinical nurse educator, "I just don't understand these comments. This nurse scored 96% on the postworkshop multiple-choice test. This nurse knew almost all the answers. We went over so many details about the culture and even provided handouts delineating the major facts." Jeannette proceeds to share the nurse's written comments with Trudy.

Nurse: "I know that cultural-specific nursing interventions can make a difference in client outcomes. I am aware that some of my patients have CVB that are different from my own. I want to become a more culturally competent nurse, so I read journal articles about culture whenever they are published in *RN* magazine. Sometimes the articles give great ideas about how to communicate appropriately with culturally different clients and even provide some understandable assessment tools. The hospital workshop on 'Meeting the Needs of Russian Immigrants' provided me with new knowledge about one of the many cultural groups that we encounter regularly at our hospital. Unfortunately, I just don't feel very confident about my abilities as a culturally competent nurse, so I don't really try to develop cultural-specific care plans or directly ask clients about their CVB. I feel as though I am prying. Besides, I might make a mistake. If culturally different clients ask me for something that isn't too extraordinary or against the usual hospital policy, I do try to accommodate them unless things get too busy."

Trudy replies, "The nurse's comments suggest that she has some cultural knowledge, cultural desire, self-awareness, conscious awareness of cultural diversity, conscious awareness of cultural incompetence, exposure to cultural assessment skills and tools, and many interactions with culturally different clients, yet lacks confidence. Cultural competence and culturally congruent care outcomes are strongly linked to confidence. Specifically, transcultural self-efficacy is the perceived confidence for performing or learning transcultural nursing skills. It is the degree to which individuals perceive they have the ability to perform the specific transcultural nursing skills needed for culturally competent and congruent care."

Trudy proceeds to share the CCC model and the TSE Pathway with Jeannette, discussing the major and minor components in each. Jeannette then recognizes that cultural competence is a multidimensional learning process that integrates transcultural skills in all three dimensions (cognitive, practical, and affective) and involves TSE (confidence) as a major influencing factor.

Based on the model, Jeannette and Trudy plan to develop future learner-centered educational experiences that (a) carefully weave cognitive, practical, and affective transcultural nursing skills; (b) encompass assessment, planning, implementation, and evaluation; and (c) integrate self-efficacy appraisals and diagnostic-specific interventions.

CHAPTER 3

A Tool for Measurement and Evaluation

- What are students' needs, values, attitudes, and skills concerning transcultural nursing?
- Which transcultural nursing skills do students perceive with more confidence?
- Which transcultural nursing skills do students perceive with less confidence?
- What are the differences in transcultural self-efficacy (TSE) perceptions between novice and advanced groups?
- What are the changes in TSE perceptions following formalized educational experiences and/or other learning experiences?
- What demographic factors influence TSE perceptions?

These underlying questions prompted the author's next level of inquiry—"How can TSE perceptions be explored, measured, and evaluated validly among novice and advanced students?" To address this question, a literature review was conducted, focusing on transcultural nursing, cultural issues, self-efficacy, learning theories, and instrumentation. The majority of self-efficacy tools described in the nursing literature pertained to client education. One self-efficacy scale, the Cultural Self-Efficacy Scale (Bernal & Froman, 1987), was designed to measure cultural self-efficacy perceptions of community health nurses within three specific client populations (black, Latino, and Southeast Asian). No self-efficacy tool had been specifically designed that would measure student's perceived self-efficacy for performing general transcultural nursing skills among clients of different cultures. Furthermore, no questionnaire had been designed for culturally diverse nursing students who must learn to care for many different groups of culturally diverse clients.

Therefore, the design of a new instrument was necessary. The author's decision to create a new instrument was further substantiated by self-efficacy theory that supports the design of detailed questionnaires (focused on specific tasks or skills) within the desired domain of inquiry (Bandura, 1982, 1989, 1997). The process of designing a new instrument included item development, item sequence, subscale sequence, expert content review, expert psychometric review, revised draft, pretest, minor revisions, and a second pretest (Jeffreys & Smodlaka, 1996). This chapter comprehensively discusses the measurement and evaluation of learners through the use of the Transcultural Self-Efficacy Tool (TSET) (see appendix A). Major components, features, and psychometric properties (reliability and validity) of the TSET are highlighted. Applied uses and evaluation strategies conclude the chapter.

TRANSCULTURAL SELF-EFFICACY TOOL DESCRIPTION

Major Components and Features

The TSET was originally designed to measure and evaluate students' confidence for performing general transcultural nursing skills among diverse populations. A generalist approach, focusing on general transcultural nursing skills, was considered most appropriate for learners without previous formal education and background in transcultural nursing, especially those who would care for clients of many different cultural backgrounds. The generalist approach emphasizes broad transcultural nursing principles, concepts, theories, and research study findings to care for clients of many different cultures (Leininger, 1989). In contrast, a specialist approach is most appropriate for learners who have mastered general transcultural nursing skills developed through formalized educational and interactive experiences. A specialist approach aims to prepare an individual as a "specialist" in one or more select cultural groups, requiring a series of specialized transcultural courses and concentrated fieldwork (Leininger, 1989; Leininger & McFarland, 2002).

Based on the literature and the results of a two-phase evaluation study (Jeffreys & Smodlaka, 1996), the 83-item TSET (Jeffreys, 1994) contains three subscales presented in the following sequence: Cognitive (25 items), Practical (30 items), and Affective (28 items). Separate subscales were created for two main reasons: (a) the most comprehensive learning includes coordinated learning in the cognitive, practical (psychomotor), and affective domains; and (b) self-efficacy theory purports that different dimensions within a specific domain of inquiry require separate subscales for accurate measurement and evaluation (Bandura, 1982, 1989). The Cognitive subscale asks respondents to rate their confidence about their knowledge concerning the ways cultural factors may influence nursing care. The Practical subscale asks respondents to rate their confidence for interviewing clients of different cultural backgrounds to learn about their values and beliefs; 30 culture-related interview topics are presented as items. Attitudes, values, and beliefs are addressed in the Affective subscale (see appendix A).

Consistent with self-efficacy measurement tool guidelines (Bandura, 1977, 1982, 1989), items are close ended and positively phrased; a 10-point rating scale from 1 (not confident) to 10 (totally confident) is used. Table 3.1 depicts the major components and features with the underlying rationale for each component and feature.

Psychometric Properties: Validity and Reliability

The author conducted a series of four studies to estimate the psychometric properties of the TSET. Psychometric properties broadly refer to the results obtained from specific statistical tests for estimating instrument validity and reliability. Results are really only estimates of the instrument's validity and reliability because a certain amount of measurement error is always present. Details about validity and reliability tests and their results are outlined in the following sections.

Validity

Validity is concerned with the accurate measurement of what an instrument is supposed to measure. For the TSET, a general question was asked: "Does the TSET accurately measure what it is supposed to measure?" To answer this broad question, three more specific questions were asked, differentiating between content validity, construct validity, and criterion-related validity.

Content validity. Content validity is concerned with whether the instrument and its items are representative of the desired content area and is best assessed by content experts (Waltz, Strickland, & Lenz, 2005; Polit & Beck, 2004). For the TSET, the question posed was "Is the TSET and its items representative of the desired content area?" The identified content area targeted the transcultural nursing skills necessary for the transcultural nurse generalist who may be caring for clients of many different cultural backgrounds. In addition, items needed to represent this content domain and be readable and appropriate for novice undergraduate nursing students. Information about the intended purpose, desired

Table 3.1 Transcultural Self-Efficacy Tool (TSET): Major Components, Features, and Rationale

TSET Description	Rationale
General Content Areas (Subscales)	
1. Cognitive	Taxonomy of educational objectives
2. Practical	(different dimensions of learning)[a]
3. Affective	Self-efficacy theory (different dimensions within a specific domain require separate subscales)[b]
Number of Items = 83	
25–30 Items on each subscale	Instrument length may affect reliability and validity[c]
Cognitive (25 items)	Select the least number of unique items to capture
Practical (30 items)	construct while avoiding redundancy[c]
Affective (28 items)	
General Item Content	
1. Specific to cultural care issues or transcultural nursing	Target purpose[d]
	Original target audience[d]
2. Appropriate for entry-level nursing students	Entry level is most basic level; therefore, items will have broader application and future use
Individual Item Content	
1. Addresses only one issue	Stimulate valid and reliable the targeted
2. Clear and succinct	population[c]
3. Avoids redundancy between items	
Item Structure	
1. Close ended	Consistent with self-efficacy theory and scales[b]
2. Positively phrased	
Rating Scale	
10-Point rating scale from 1 (not confident) to 10 (totally confident)	Bandura's use of 10-point scales[b]
	More discriminating than 6-point rating scale[d]
Item Sequence	
1. Clustering items sequentially as they occur (e.g., pregnancy, birth).	Psychometric guidelines[c]
	Taxonomy for affective objectives[a]
2. Least stressful to more stressful or complex	Self-efficacy theory and scales[b,e,f]
Emphasis on Individual Efficacy Appraisal	
1. Personalized items and directions using second pronoun	Psychometric guidelines[c]
	Increase reliability and validity of responses[c]
2. Highlighting and underlining important words	
Subscale Sequence	
1. Cognitive	Prevents anchoring effect as supported by pretesting
2. Practical	various forms of TSET subscale sequence[d]
3. Affective	

[a]From Bloom, B.S., Englehart, M.D., Furst, E.J., Hill, W.H., & Krath Wohl, D.R. (1956); Harrow (1972); Krathwohl, Bloom, and Masia (1964).
[b]From Bandura (1977, 1982, 1986, 1989).
[c]From Sudman and Bradburn (1991).
[d]From Jeffreys and Smodlaka (1996).
[e] From Cervone and Peake (1986).
[f] From Cervone & Palmer (1990).

content area, and self-efficacy theory was distributed to the content experts. Content validity was established by six doctoral-prepared nurses certified in transcultural nursing (Jeffreys & Smodlaka, 1996).

Construct validity. Assessment of construct validity evaluates the degree to which a tool measures the construct being studied. Construct validation attempts to validate the tool's underlying theoretical concepts and proposed relationships between the concepts (Munro, 2005; Polit & Beck, 2004). An instrument whose performance is consistent with the underlying conceptual expectations demonstrates adequate construct validity (Carmines & Zeller, 1979). To answer the question "To what degree does the TSET measure TSE?" both a contrasted group approach and a factor analysis were conducted.

Two studies used the contrasted group approach for estimating construct validity and addressed the question "Are mean scores on the TSET significantly different between two contrasted groups (novice students and advanced students)?" Consistent findings from a longitudinal study and a cross-sectional study supported that the TSET detected differences in TSE perceptions within groups and between groups on all subscales (Jeffreys, 2000; Jeffreys & Smodlaka, 1999a, 1999b). Several underlying theoretical assumptions were supported in these studies:

- TSE is a dynamic construct that changes over time and is influenced by formalized exposure to culture care concepts (transcultural nursing).
- Learners are most confident about their attitudes (affective dimension) and least confident about their transcultural nursing knowledge (cognitive dimension).
- Novice learners will have lower self-efficacy perceptions than advanced learners.
- The greatest change in TSE perceptions will be detected in individuals with low self-efficacy (low confidence) initially, who have then been exposed to formalized transcultural nursing concepts and experiences.

Next, the factor analysis study evaluated the degree to which individual items clustered around one or more conceptual dimension. Items that cluster together (to become a "factor") should make sense conceptually, thus supporting the underlying conceptual framework and attesting to the construct validity of the instrument. The factor analysis study (Jeffreys & Smodlaka, 1998) broadly explored "What is the factor composition of the TSET?"

Several different statistical procedures may be employed in factor analysis. Each procedure contains certain errors or assumptions; therefore, all factor analysis options were appraised. Review of statistical theory and collaboration with a psychometric expert guided the decision-making process. The first step of factor analysis begins with a matrix of correlation coefficients between items (Comrey, 1973; Munro, 2005). Items should contribute uniquely and satisfactorily to the instrument, avoiding any redundancy between items. Generally, items that correlate below 0.30 are not sufficiently related and therefore do not contribute to the construct's measurement; items that correlate above 0.70 are considered redundant and unnecessary (Ferketich, 1991). The question "Do all items on the TSET contribute uniquely and sufficiently to the TSE construct?" was evaluated via an interitem correlation matrix. All items correlated between 0.30 and 0.70; therefore, it was assumed that all TSET items contributed uniquely and sufficiently to the TSE construct (Jeffreys, 2000; Jeffreys & Smodlaka, 1998).

The next issue pertained to the assessment of intercorrelations between the three subscales. Within self-efficacy theory, separate subscales should be designed to measure the distinct dimensions within a domain of inquiry. In the assessment of self-efficacy, intercorrelations between subscales corroborate that each subscale measures different dimensions within the domain (Bandura, 1989). To answer the question "Are the Cognitive, Practical, and Affective subscales correlated with each other?" subscale means were compared. Intercorrelations between subscales were statistically significant and ranged from 0.53 (Cognitive and Affective) to 0.62 (Cognitive and Practical) and 0.68 (Practical and Affective). These results helped validate the following assumptions in the underlying framework:

- Learning in the cognitive, practical, and affective dimensions is paradoxically distinct, yet interrelated.
- Learners are most confident about their attitudes (affective dimension) and least confident about their transcultural nursing knowledge (cognitive dimension).

Factor analysis studies are sometimes used for determining parsimony through item deletion, meaning that items that do not load on a factor are deleted to make the instrument shorter. Using conventional procedures for factor analysis as reported in the literature (Gilley & Uhlig, 1993; Kim & Mueller, 1978; Nunnally & Bernstein, 1994), a principal component analysis with the varimax rotation yielded a nine-factor structure for the study sample (Jeffreys, 2000; Jeffreys & Smodlaka, 1998). With factor loadings set at 0.50, 70 items loaded on the nine factors;

none of the 70 items loaded significantly on any other factor. "All nine factors had eigenvalues greater than 1.00, accounted for 62% of the total variance, and contained at least three items whose difference in loading on the other factors was greater than .30" (Jeffreys & Smodlaka, 1998, p. 223). The question "Should any items be dropped?" was considered. Because dropping items after just one factor analysis study should be viewed cautiously (Comrey, 1973) and because the interitem correlation matrix indicated that each item contributed uniquely and significantly to the TSE construct, no items were dropped. Future factor analysis studies with large samples will provide greater guidance as to whether items should be deleted.

Factors derived from an analysis provide one interpretation of the data and are useful for understanding relationships within a specific domain; however, the interpretation should be confirmed with other types of evidence (Comrey, 1973). In addition, construct validation should focus on the degree to which an instrument is consistent with the related literature and underlying conceptual framework (Carmines & Zeller, 1979); therefore, this was also examined. For the TSET, supporting evidence included several key theoretical issues. First, the factors related to the literature in transcultural nursing and the underlying conceptual framework. Items that clustered together made sense conceptually and were accordingly labeled: recognition, kinship and social factors, professional nursing care, cultural background and identity, life cycle transitional phenomena, awareness of cultural gap, communication, self-awareness, and appreciation (Jeffreys, 2000; Jeffreys & Smodlaka, 1998). Second, items that clustered together were from the same subscale, clustering exclusively on the Cognitive, Practical, or Affective subscale (see appendices B, C, and D). Subscale exclusivity most likely implies that within each broad educational category, as captured in the three TSET subscales, there are several underlying theoretical dimensions that contribute to the TSE construct (Jeffreys & Smodlaka, 1998). Third, students were most confident about Affective subscale factors and least confident about Cognitive subscale factors. Fourth, changes in mean scores on each of the nine factors occurred in the expected direction for novice and advanced students (means were higher for advanced students on all factors).

Results from this phase of the factor analysis study helped validate the following assumptions:

- Learning in the cognitive, practical, and affective dimensions is paradoxically distinct, yet interrelated.
- Learners are most confident about their attitudes (affective dimension) and least confident about their transcultural nursing knowledge (cognitive dimension).

- Novice learners will have lower self-efficacy perceptions than advanced learners.

Criterion-related validity. Another important consideration pertains to the assessment of criterion-related validity. Criterion-related validity examines the degree to which the subject's performance on the measurement tool and the subject's actual behavior are related (LoBiondo-Wood & Haber, 1998; Polit & Beck, 2004). In other words, criterion related validity addresses "How is performance on a measurement tool and actual behavior related?" and may be assessed using different approaches. For the TSET, predictive validity was examined. Predictive validity examines the degree of correlation between the measure of the concept and a future measure of the same concept. An underlying theoretical assumption was that TSE is a dynamic construct that changes over time and is influenced by formalized exposure to culture care concepts (transcultural nursing). The question "Does the TSET measure changes in TSE after formalized exposure to transcultural nursing?" was most directly addressed in a longitudinal study. Results indicated statistically significant differences in TSE perceptions between the first and fourth clinical semester (Jeffreys & Smodlaka, 1999a). The greatest changes were detected in students with lower self-efficacy initially who had then been exposed to a 2-year educational experience that integrated transcultural nursing concepts, issues, and skills within theory and clinical work. In a cross-sectional study, TSE scores also demonstrated changes in the expected (predicted) direction. Demographic variables (age, gender, income, ethnicity, and racial group identity) did not influence TSE perceptions or the types of changes in TSE perceptions (Jeffreys & Smodlaka, 1999b). The results supported the following underlying assumptions:

- TSE is a dynamic construct that changes over time and is influenced by formalized exposure to culture care concepts (transcultural nursing).
- Learners are most confident about their attitudes (affective dimension) and least confident about their transcultural nursing knowledge (cognitive dimension).
- All students and nurses (regardless of age, ethnicity, gender, sexual orientation, lifestyle, religion, socioeconomic status, geographic location, or race) require formalized educational experiences to meet culture care needs of diverse individuals.
- Novice learners will have lower self-efficacy perceptions than advanced learners.
- The greatest change in TSE perceptions will be detected in individuals with low self-efficacy (low confidence) initially, who have

then been exposed to formalized transcultural nursing concepts and experiences.

Predictive validity is also concerned with the degree to which an individual's performance on the questionnaire correlates with a predetermined outcome behavior. The desired outcome behavior is a high level of cultural competent behaviors resulting in culturally congruent care; however; the evaluation of cultural competency in the clinical setting is complex. The potential for changed behaviors with known observations, confounded by the limited availability of qualified observers and valid measurement strategies, presents challenges for directly estimating predictions of TSE on actual behavior. According to Bandura's (1986) theory, resilient (strong) self-efficacy perceptions result in higher levels of goal commitment, motivation, persistence, learning, and skill performance. Commitment and motivation are essential components in achieving cultural competency (Campinha-Bacote, 1999, 2003; Chang, 1995); therefore. it can only be assumed that TSE perceptions will directly influence cultural competency through commitment and motivation. Other studies indicated that self-efficacy is a mediator of commitment and motivation, thereby affecting outcome behaviors (Bandura, 1996a, 1996b, 1997; Bandura & Schunk, 1981; Lent, Lopez, & Bieschke, 1993; Mone, Baker, & Jeffries, 1995; Saks, 1995).

Reliability

An instrument cannot be valid without demonstrated reliability. *Reliability* refers to the degree of accuracy and consistency in measurement. Reliability examines the extent to which an instrument provides the same results on repeated uses (LoBiondo-Wood & Haber, 1998; Polit & Beck, 2004).

Usually reliability tests are performed each time the instrument is used because instrument reliability is population specific rather than an inherent instrument property (Nunnally & Bernstein, 1994). With the TSET, the broad question concerning reliability asked, "To what extent does the TSET provide the same results on repeated uses with different samples?" To answer this question, two more specific questions were asked to differentiate between internal consistency and stability.

Internal consistency. Internal consistency is concerned with the degree to which questionnaire items correlate with each other and reflect the same concept. High levels of internal consistency in the total instrument and within its subscales permit tallying of items for the purpose of scoring and data analysis (LoBiondo-Wood & Haber, 1998; Nunnally &

Bernstein, 1994). The question "To what degree are items on the TSET internally consistent?" could also be phrased to ask "To what degree do TSET items correlate with each other and reflect the same construct?" Another important question "Is the internal consistency of the TSET adequate?" necessitated comprehension of methodological guidelines concerning minimal adequacy results. Reliability tests are reported as reliability coefficients. Perfectly correlated items would be demonstrated by a coefficient of 1.00. Generally, a reliability coefficient of 0.70 is considered acceptable for new instruments. In contrast, a minimum reliability coefficient of 0.80 is considered adequate for well-established instruments (Nunnally & Bernstein, 1994).

These questions led to two approaches for reliability testing: Cronbach's alpha (coefficient alpha) and split-half reliability. Cronbach's alpha is the preferred measure of internal consistency because all items are compared with each other and with the total questionnaire. In split-half reliability, one half of the instrument or subscale is compared with the other half. This approach is less accurate and often yields lower results (Nunnally & Bernstein, 1994). Consistent with this methodological assumption, split-half reliability results on the total TSET and its subscales were lower, ranging from 0.76 to 0.92. Cronbach's alpha was calculated across several studies, each time yielding coefficient alpha ranging from 0.92 to 0.98 on the total TSET instrument and its subscales (Jeffreys, 2000). In addition, alpha coefficients ranged from 0.87 to 0.95 when testing for the internal consistency of items within each of the identified nine factors (Jeffreys, 2000; Jeffreys & Smodlaka, 1998). The results indicated that the TSET had high estimates of reliability (internal consistency) and supported the use of subscale scoring to measure the various dimensions of TSE perceptions.

Stability. Stability aims to measure whether the measurement of the construct is stable and addresses "To what degree will the same results be obtained on repeated instrument administrations?" One desired use of the TSET was to detect TSE perceptual changes over time; therefore, it was essential to use the test–retest method for assessing stability. Consistent with recommended protocols for test–retest methodology (Carmines & Zeller, 1979; Nunnally & Bernstein, 1994), a 2-week interval between TSET administrations was selected. Specifically, the test–retest method explored "To what degree will the same results be obtained on two administrations of the TSET following a 2-week interval?", "To what degree is the TSET stable?", and "Is the stability of the TSET adequate?"

Because test–retest reliability is considered the least conclusive measure of reliability, it was anticipated that results would be lower than with the split-half or Cronbach's alpha methods. Test–retest correlation

Table 3.2 Summary of Transcultural Self-Efficacy Tool (TSET) Reliability Tests and Results (Jeffreys, 2000)

Type Assessed	Method	Results
Internal consistency	Cronbach's alpha	0.92–0.98
	Split-half	0.76–0.92
Stability	Test–retest	0.63–0.75

coefficients for the total TSET ranged from 0.63 to 0.75, suggesting moderate stability. However, it should be noted that lower values may actually signify that the trait changes over time independent of the instrument's stability (Carmines & Zeller, 1979). It is possible to surmise that students' exposure to multidimensional learning experiences via assignments, classroom, and clinical settings over 2 weeks could make a slight positive difference. Table 3.2 summarizes TSET reliability results in the initial instrument studies (Jeffreys & Smodlaka, 1996, 1998, 1999a, 1999b).

Scoring

As mentioned previously, the high levels of internal consistency within the whole TSET instrument and within each subscale supported the use of scores for data analyses. Bandura (1986) recommended assessing both the strength and magnitude (level) of self-efficacy. A review of literature by Lee and Bobko (1994) identified five different ways of operationalizing self-efficacy based on Bandura's recommendations. Consistent with many other self-efficacy instruments (Bandura, 1989; Berry, West, & Dennehey, 1989; Brown, Lent, & Larkin, 1989; Cervone, 1989; Hackett, 1985; Lent, Brown, & Larkin, 1986, 1987; Shell, Murphy, & Bruning, 1989), scoring of the TSET includes subscale calculations of self-efficacy strength (SEST) and self-efficacy level (SEL). SEST refers to the average strength of self-efficacy perceptions within a particular dimension (subscale) of the construct. On the TSET, SEST scores are calculated by totaling subscale item responses and dividing by the number of subscale items, resulting in the mean score (see Table 3.3). SEST scores are used most often in self-efficacy studies (Lee & Bobko, 1994) (see appendix E).

SEL refers to the number of items perceived at a specified minimum level of confidence. In studies with phobics and low academic achievers, SEL has been used to identify individuals with "low efficacy" and then track SEL changes following treatment interventions. Individuals with less than 20% confidence are inefficacious and are at high risk for avoidance behaviors and severe stress (Bandura, 1977, 1982; Bandura & Schunk, 1981). Although this benchmark has been used with phobics and

Table 3.3 Self-Efficacy Strength (SEST) Score Calculation: Subscale Mean

	Cognitive Subscale	Practical Subscale	Affective Subscale
Formula			
$\dfrac{\text{Item Response Sum}}{\text{No. of Subscale Items}}$	$\dfrac{\text{Add Item Responses}}{25}$	$\dfrac{\text{Add Item Responses}}{30}$	$\dfrac{\text{Add Item Responses}}{28}$
Application	$\dfrac{140}{25}$	$\dfrac{210}{30}$	$\dfrac{220}{28}$
	SEST = 5.6	SEST = 7.0	SEST = 7.9

academic low achievers, it has been adjusted in samples where greater self-efficacy perceptions have been anticipated. For example, Bandura and Schunk (1981) raised the benchmark to 40%, reflecting a "moderate degree of assurance" (p. 594). Some self-efficacy studies have not included the evaluation of SEL (Lee & Bobko, 1994). Other researchers have noted redundancy between the two measures and have chosen to only report one measure (score) of self-efficacy (Cervone, 1989).

On the TSET, SEL initially referred to the number of subscale items students perceived with more than 20% confidence; however, the 20% benchmark may need to be raised in samples where greater self-efficacy perceptions are observed, desirable, and/or expected (see Table 3.4). For SEL scores to be meaningful, they must discriminate within the sample. If the benchmark is too low for the sample, then most (or even all) of

Table 3.4 Self-Efficacy Level (SEL) Score Calculation: Sample Methods

	Cognitive Subscale	Practical Subscale	Affective Subscale
Sample 1			
SEL = total no. of item responses with greater than 20% confidence	Total No. of Items with Scores ≥ 3	Total No. of Items with Scores ≥ 3	Total No. of Items with Scores ≥ 3
Application	22 items ≥ 3 SEL = 22	28 items ≥ 3 SEL = 28	28 items ≥ 3 SEL = 28
Sample 2			
SEL = total no. of item responses with at least 40% confidence	Total No. of Items with Scores ≥ 4	Total No. of Items with Scores ≥ 4	Total No. of Items with Scores ≥ 4
Application	17 items ≥ 4 SEL = 17	20 items ≥ 4 SEL = 20	24 items ≥ 4 SEL = 24

the sample will have the same SEL score. For example, in several studies, the 20% SEL benchmark resulted in few students (Jeffreys & Smodlaka, 1999a, 1999b; Lim et al., 2004; MacQuarrie, 2004) and few nurses (Dolgan, 2001; Toney, 2004; Velez, 2005) who did not meet the 20% benchmark. Future studies may want to raise the benchmark standards, especially if the overall goal is to enhance cultural competence and provide high levels of culturally congruent care to culturally diverse patients.

Both SEST and SEL scores can be calculated to grasp the multidimensional nature of TSE. These scores provide valuable but different information in understanding initial TSE perceptions. Tracking changes over time and/or following an educational intervention can monitor both SEST and SEL. SEST scores present the average score; therefore, low or high item responses may be hidden within the average (mean). SEST and SEL scores can be used to detect changes over time, compare with a demographic variable, or compare within the group.

Grouping samples into low, medium, and high efficacy groups based on SEST, SEL, and/or some other criterion permits further comparative analyses and the identification of at-risk individuals (inefficacious or supremely efficacious). Inefficacious individuals are at risk for avoiding tasks; supremely efficacious (overly confident) individuals are at risk because of inadequate preparation and/or viewing the task as unimportant (Bandura, 1982).

Several different methods may be used for group categorization and comparison; several sample methods are proposed in appendix F; however, future studies are needed to assess validation. The study purpose and sample may guide method selection for group categorization. For example, coding may occur in the following manner: (a) low (students who select a 1 or 2 response on 80% or more of the subscale items); (b) high (students who select a 9 or 10 response on 80% or more of the subscale items; and (c) medium (students who select a 3 through 8 response on 80% or more of the subscale items or who do not fall into the low or high group) (Dolgan, 2001; Jeffreys & Smodlaka, 1999a, 1999b; Lim et al., 2004; MacQuarrie, 2004; Toney, 2004; Velez, 2005). Alternatively (in samples with few 1 or 2 responses/subscale), respondents with any 1 or 2 responses may be categorized as low SEL, if adhering to the proposed 20% confidence benchmark indicating "low" or "at risk." The definition of the "high" group could be "respondents who selected 9 and 10 responses for all subscale items." Here, the medium group would constitute respondents who did not fall into the other two groups. In other samples (especially where low self-efficacy perceptions can be anticipated to be less prevalent), still other techniques may be employed for grouping. For example, the 20% benchmark for SEL could be raised to 40% (Bandura & Schunk, 1981). Another approach involves percentages or standard deviations to compute low, middle, and high groups. For example, the medium group can be defined as plus or minus one standard deviation from the subscale mean. Respondents below this criterion would be labeled "low"; respondents above this criterion would constitute the "high" group. Further research is needed to appraise various approaches.

In summary, SEST scores are most often used in self-efficacy studies (Lee & Bobko, 1994). Calculation of SEST scores for each of the TSET subscales is routinely recommended whenever the TSET is used. TSET SEL scores are an additional, supplemental approach for analyzing data. Different methods can be employed to group individuals into low efficacy, medium efficacy, and high efficacy groups for the purpose of identifying at-risk individuals and tracking changes.

EVALUATING TRANSCULTURAL SELF-EFFICACY PERCEPTIONS

Although the TSET was specifically designed to measure and evaluate undergraduate nursing students' confidence for performing general transcultural nursing skills among diverse populations, nurse researchers have requested the TSET for use with graduate students and/or for use with nurses working in various clinical agencies. Researchers in other health professions worldwide have requested the TSET for review and possible use, adaptation, and/or translation. Because the TSET does not selectively target specific cultural groups, but rather it broadly asks respondents to consider general principles related to culturally different clients, it has broader application among culturally diverse health care professionals who provide care for many culturally diverse clients. The generalist approach (as emphasized in the TSET) was considered most appropriate for learners without previous formal education and background in transcultural nursing and/or the transcultural nurse generalist who will provide care for clients of many different cultural backgrounds.

One underlying assumption of the TSET is that all students and nurses (regardless of age, ethnicity, gender, sexual orientation, lifestyle, religion, socioeconomic status, geographic location, or race) require formalized educational experiences to meet culture care needs of diverse individuals. (The same assumption applies across other health professional disciplines.)

Unfortunately, the numbers of nurses and other health professionals who have received formal education experiences in transcultural topics and cultural competence are few (Andrews, 1995; Leininger, 1995b; Leininger & McFarland, 2002; Wilson & Houghtaling, 2001). Only relatively recently have accrediting agencies, professional organizations, journals, textbooks, and films, included culture and culturally congruent care as an essential dimension in achieving quality health outcomes. Therefore, it is reasonable to assume that an instrument that is readable and appropriate for novice undergraduate students may also be appropriate for other populations; however, only trial use and ongoing instrument evaluation will provide definitive information.

Usability may be applicable to populations who have had little or no formalized education experiences in transcultural nursing and cultural competence and/or those without opportunities for field application/interaction with culturally different clients and/or nurses/health professionals. Usability may also extend to populations who have had formal and/or informal exposure to transcultural nursing, culturally different clients, and culturally different health care professional colleagues. For example, Toney (2004) used the TSET to measure TSE among community health nurses who frequently encounter culturally diverse clients in their clinical practice. Within the hospital setting, educators have used the TSET as a pretest, posttest, and guide for future cultural competence education planning. For example, Dolgan (2001), Platter (2005), and Velez (2005) reported changes in nurses' TSE perceptions following educational interventions. Within the discipline of medicine, the TSET has been adapted for use with physicians in Australia (Shadbolt, 2004). Ultimately, it is the study purpose, design, research questions/hypotheses, and sample that must guide a researcher's decision to use the TSET. Future research with the TSET among similar and different populations will expand knowledge concerning TSE and the TSET.

Evaluation of TSE perceptions may be used for various purposes targeting the individual and/or groups (Box 3.1). The purposes are to

- Develop a composite/baseline of learners' needs, values, attitudes, and skills concerning transcultural nursing (or health care).
- Identify general transcultural skills perceived with more confidence (or those as less difficult or stressful).
- Identify general transcultural skills perceived with less confidence (or those as more difficult or stressful).
- Identify differences within groups.
- Identify differences between groups.
- Identify at-risk individuals (low confidence or overly confident).
- Evaluate the effectiveness of specific teaching interventions.
- Assess changes in TSE perceptions over time.

Although self-report instruments present certain limitations, the construct of self-efficacy can only be evaluated by self-appraisal and self-report (Bandura, 1996a, 1996b, 1997). Choice of a valid and reliable instrument will help decrease the limitations associated with measurement error and increase the confidence with which researchers interpret data. Using the TSET, several different approaches can be implemented to yield valuable information necessary to guide future research, education, and practice. The selected approach will be determined by the study purpose, design, research questions/hypotheses, sample, and researcher. Ongoing instrument evaluation must be an integral component in every study. Comparison of SEST scores, SEL scores, groups (low, medium, high), individual item responses, and factor mean scores can be used to answer research questions/hypotheses. Collection of appropriate and relevant demographic data will be valuable in interpreting findings and may be useful for descriptive or inferential statistical analyses. (Appendices F and G present examples of demographic data potentially relevant for collection with the TSET.) Researchers' examination of the results in relation to the proposed underlying assumptions of the CCC model can further substantiate the proposed theoretical assumptions. For example, among various study samples, respondents are most confident about their affective skills and least confident about their knowledge (Dolgan, 2001; Jeffreys, 2000; Jeffreys & Smodlaka, 1996, 1998, 1999a, 1999b; Lim et al., 2004; MacQuarrie, 2004; Platter, 2005; Toney, 2004; Velez, 2005; Wilson & Houghtaling, 2001). Strategies for interpreting learners' TSE perceptions with implications for cultural competence education are discussed in chapter 4.

KEY POINT SUMMARY

- Based on the literature and the results of a two-phase evaluation study, the 83-item TSET was designed to measure and evaluate students' confidence for performing general transcultural nursing skills among diverse populations.
- The process of designing the TSET included item development, item sequence, subscale sequence, expert content review, expert psychometric review, revised draft, pretest, minor revisions, and a second pretest.
- The TSET contains three subscales presented in the following sequence: Cognitive (25 items), Practical (30 items), and Affective (28 items).
- The Cognitive subscale asks respondents to rate their confidence about their knowledge concerning the ways cultural factors may influence nursing care.
- The Practical subscale asks respondents to rate their confidence for interviewing clients of different cultural backgrounds to learn

about their values and beliefs; 30 culture-related interview topics are presented as items.

- Attitudes, values, and beliefs are addressed in the Affective subscale.
- Validity tests addressed content validity, criterion-related validity, and construct validity.
- Consistent findings from a longitudinal study and a cross-sectional study supported that the TSET detected differences in TSE perceptions within groups and between groups on all subscales.
- A factor analysis study yielded nine factors: recognition, kinship and social factors, professional nursing care, cultural background and identity, life cycle transitional phenomena, awareness of cultural gap, communication, self-awareness, and appreciation. Items clustered exclusively on the Cognitive, Practical, or Affective subscale.
- Reliability tests for internal consistency and stability indicated adequate reliability.
- Scoring on the TSET includes subscales SEST and SEL.
- Several different methods may be employed for grouping respondents into low, medium, and high efficacy (confidence) groups.
- Comparison of SEST scores, SEL scores, groups (low, medium, high), individual item responses, and factor mean scores can be used to answer specific research questions/hypotheses. The selected approach will be determined by the study purpose, design, research questions/hypotheses, sample, and researcher.
- The TSET has been used in grant-funded projects and studies and has been requested by graduate students, faculty, and health care professionals in various disciplines from around the world.

Box 3.1   Educator-in-Action Vignette

Professor Quest becomes interested in exploring, measuring, and evaluating undergraduate students' baseline self-efficacy perceptions prior to the design and implementation of educational interventions to develop cultural competence. He plans to systematically re-evaluate self-efficacy perceptions following the implementation of educational interventions. Following a literature review, Professor Quest contemplates the use of the TSET to explore baseline TSE perceptions, conduct follow-up measures of TSE after educational interventions are introduced into the curriculum, and evaluate changes within the three dimensions of learning.

He decides to pilot the TSET with a small group of approximately 30 first-semester students. After obtaining permission to use the TSET (see appendix I), Professor Quest prepares a "Pilot Test Worksheet" to guide evaluation of the

TSET for use with his prospective larger study (see Table 3.5). Based on the pilot test results, he decides to use the TSET in a larger, multisite study to explore beginning students' baseline perceptions before any formal exposure to transcultural nursing educational interventions.

To further explore construct validity and to identify target area clusters that may require priority educational interventions based on lowest confidence ratings, Professor Quest plans to explore the factorial composition of the TSET. Comparison of his results with previous TSET factor analysis study findings, the related literature, and the underlying conceptual framework will expand scientific knowledge and guide future research and educational innovations. After designing and implementing transcultural nursing educational interventions (see chapter 5 for examples), the TSET will be readministered to and evaluated for changes in TSE. Comparisons will include SEST (subscale mean scores), SEL, and groups (low, medium, and high). Early collaboration with a statistician assists Professor Quest in the decision-making process and plan for statistical analysis.

Table 3.5   Pilot Test Worksheet

	Cognitive	Practical	Affective	Total TSET
Completion Time				X
Item responses				
Range	X	X	X	
Mode	X	X	X	
Median	X	X	X	
Frequency (each item option)	X	X	X	
Subscale Mean (SEST)	X	X	X	
Subscale SEL				
20% Benchmark	X	X	X	
30% Benchmark	X	X	X	
40% Benchmark	X	X	X	
Reliability Tests				
Cronbach's alpha	X	X	X	X
Split-half	X	X	X	X
Validity Tests				
Construct (hypothesis testing approach): students will be least confident about their knowledge and most confident about their attitudes, values, and beliefs	Are SEST scores lowest?	Are SEST scores neither highest nor lowest?	Are SEST scores highest?	

CHAPTER 4

A Guide for Interpreting Learners' Perceptions, Identifying At-Risk Individuals, and Avoiding Pitfalls

Empirical support for self-efficacy as a predictor of cultural competence is more difficult to establish than conceptually acknowledging that self-efficacy perceptions play a vital role in cultural competence development and culturally congruent care actions. Theoretical background information must be carefully considered when interpreting findings and demonstrating empirical support. For example, the CCC model (see Figure 2.1) illustrates the proposed connections between the foundational concepts. Chapter 2 details major components underlying the conceptual model, incorporating the main theoretical tenets of Bandura's self-efficacy theory (Bandura, 1982, 1986, 1989, 1997). Finally, Figure 2.2 depicts the directional pathways involved in TSE, cultural competence development, and culturally congruent care actions, further expanding on theoretical background information.

Because the evaluation of self-efficacy relies on respondents' self-perceptions, there will always be some error associated with self-report measures; however, the only way that self-efficacy can be measured is with a self-report measurement tool. Despite the limitations that self-report measurement tools present, efforts can be made to increase the usability and interpretation of results by using a valid measurement tool and by customizing various steps and components of the research process to appropriately complement each other. Avoiding pitfalls in the initial research design will improve the interpretation of findings. Similarly, avoiding pit-falls in the interpretation of findings will enhance the study's validity and future usability and generalizability.

Making sense of transcultural self-efficacy (TSE) perceptions is a key component in this interpretive process. This chapter guides educators in the interpretation of TSE perceptions and in avoiding pitfalls in research design and interpretation. The identification of at-risk individuals through the interpretation of findings is highlighted.

INTERPRETATION

Making sense of TSE perceptions must be grounded in self-efficacy theory. A quick overview of essential theoretical elements will aid in interpreta-tion. One must know what to look for, what data findings suggest, and how to subsequently formulate valid empirical conclusions. Several main theoretical features emphasizing connections to data interpretation are presented.

A key concept in Bandura's (1986) social cognitive theory is that learning and motivation for learning is directly influenced by self-efficacy perceptions. Self-efficacy perceptions are domain and task specific. Indi-viduals with strong self-efficacy perceptions in a specific domain think, feel, and act differently from those who are inefficacious or those who are overly confident. Therefore, when interpreting findings, one will look for ways to differentiate between individuals who demon-strate strong (resilient) self-efficacy, low self-efficacy (inefficacious), or supremely high self-efficacy (overconfidence). For example, TSE percep-tions as measured by the Transcultural Self-Efficacy Tool (TSET) can be differentiated by SEST scores, SEL scores, comparison of factor mean scores, and/or grouping into low, medium, and high groups based on the selected grouping methodology. See chapter 3 for details on the TSET.

Strong (resilient) self-efficacy enhances sociocognitive functioning in several ways: (a) new or difficult tasks are viewed as challenges that are accepted willingly; (b) great preparatory efforts are exhibited; (c) strong goal commitment and persistence behaviors are enhanced; (d) failures and setbacks are attributed to insufficient effort; and (e) more energy is expended to overcome failures, hardships, setbacks, and potential stres-sors in an effort to achieve goals (Bandura, 1986). A strong (resilient) self-efficacy to withstand failures combined with some uncertainty (task perceived as a challenge rather than self-doubts about capability) will encourage preparatory efforts and thus enhance performance outcomes (Bandura, 1982, 1989). It is presumed that such individuals are highly motivated and actively seek help to maximize their transcultural nursing skills and cultural competence development. Based on the proposed pathways (see Figure 2.2), resilient individuals would be the most likely to persist in cultural competence development and the most likely to achieve culturally congruent care actions.

At-Risk Individuals

In contrast, the inefficacious individual (one with low confidence levels) is at risk for lowered persistence, motivation, and goal commitment. He or she may give up when obstacles or hardships are encountered. Such individuals may easily become discouraged if they do not quickly grasp new concepts, skills, or knowledge. That is, they may view transcultural learning tasks as overwhelming and insurmountable obstacles, threats, and hardships to be avoided. Consequently, decreased effort may be engaged, and lowered persistence with transcultural nursing skills may ensue. Low self-efficacy can affect cultural competence development directly, if individuals quit without even trying and then avoid cultural assessments, or indirectly, through poor nursing outcomes and/or through negative psychological outcomes. Poor nursing outcomes (achievement of negative client health outcomes) may be caused by culturally incongruent care. Such individuals become increasingly overwhelmed, focused on failure, dissatisfied, and stressed (see Figure 2.2).

Interpretation of data to identify inefficacious individuals is therefore crucial. In addition, individuals with low self-efficacy benefit the most with diagnostic specific interventions designed to enhance self-efficacy and other academic and psychological outcomes (Brown et al., 1989; Jeffreys & Smodlaka, 1999a; Lent et al., 1987; Zimmerman, 1995). Early identification of inefficacious students followed by diagnostic-prescriptive interventions can help students maximize strengths, minimize weakness, and facilitate success (Jeffreys, 1993, 2000, 2004; Jeffreys & Smodlaka, 1998, 1999a, 1999b). Because inefficacious individuals often lose motivation and are reluctant to actively seek assistance, the educator plays a key role in initiating actions with inefficacious individuals. (The broad term *educator* is used to describe any qualified individual in the position to provide transcultural educational interventions. Examples include qualified nursing faculty, clinical educators, preceptors, nurse managers, mentors, certified transcultural nurses, and nursing organizational leaders.) Although self-efficacy appraisal is task specific, repeated failures and negative psychological outcomes decrease self-efficacy for learning and performing the necessary tasks for becoming a culturally competent registered nurse, thereby lowering persistence and commitment behaviors overall.

Other at-risk individuals are those who are supremely efficacious (overly confident). Supremely efficacious individuals may be totally unaware of their weaknesses, underestimate the task or its importance, overlook the task, overestimate their abilities, and overrate their strengths (Bandura, 1982). Consequently, overly confident individuals may not see the need for adequate preparation, restructuring of priorities, or time management to accommodate transcultural tasks. Therefore, such individuals may not be adequately prepared. Cultural competency development is affected indirectly through poor skill outcomes and negative psychological outcomes. Poor, weak, or unsuccessful performances can lead to feeling overwhelmed, surprised or shocked, dissatisfied, and stress. Unfortunately, some supremely efficacious individuals may not even be aware that cultural incongruent care actions have adversely impacted a client's emotional and physical health outcomes.

Because supremely efficacious individuals often lack motivation for the task and see no need to seek assistance, the educator plays a key role in initiating actions with overly confident individuals. Early identification of supremely efficacious individuals can help individuals realistically appraise one's strengths and weaknesses and recognize the need for adequate preparation for the achievement of successful outcomes. Because students (especially beginning students) may not know what to expect in nursing, students may need much guidance in ongoing self-appraisal. Realistic self-efficacy appraisal allows one to seek action to enhance strengths and remedy weaknesses. Unfortunately, supremely efficacious individuals may not be restricted to beginning students but may encompass nurses and other health care professionals at various career stages.

Curricular Appraisal

Although the identification of at-risk individuals followed by teaching interventions is one proposed purpose of interpreting self-efficacy perceptions, interpretation may also be done to guide curricular innovations. For example, if first-semester baccalaureate nursing students complete the TSET and consistently report lower confidence for five particular items on the Cognitive subscale, this flags that these empirical finding should be further explored. Soliciting qualitative comments may add richness to the data and allow greater insight. Examining the first-semester nursing course in relation to these items/topics may uncover an educational gap, suggesting supplementary educational strategies to enhance transcultural nursing skills specifically to these topics. Yet, if it makes sense that first-semester students would have lower confidence for a cluster of items, then this helps validate the measurement tool and lends greater support for overall study results. For example, if students report lower confidence for topics not covered in the current course or in any previous courses, it makes conceptual sense that students would have lower confidence. However, if students just completed a course focused on maternal and child health, yet reported lower confidence for TSET Cognitive subscale items "pregnancy," "birth," and "growth and development," there would be cause for concern. Exploring underlying course and curricular objectives and desired outcomes would be necessary. Using a longitudinal study design will permit the examination of within-group changes over time, providing data on the impact of subsequent courses and other educational experiences throughout the curriculum.

AVOIDING PITFALLS

As with all data interpretation, but especially with data involving self-report measurement tools and the measurement of constructs that are difficult to measure, data interpretation must be viewed cautiously. Interpretation must be realistic. An overconfident or inefficacious approach to data interpretation should be avoided because both approaches can interfere with the best interpretation that will have the most practical significance and usability. Consciously recognizing study limitations and avoiding overgeneralization of results will help keep overconfidence in check. Acknowledging the positive findings rather than negating all results because of slight imperfections in study design or other limitations is another consideration. Recognizing that statistically insignificant results can have practical significance and recognizing that statistically significant results do not always yield meaningful findings or practical significance are equally important. The following sections discuss strategies for avoiding pitfalls in research design and interpretation.

Recognize Limitations Related to Measurement Level

Self-efficacy measurement tools are reported to provide data at the ordinal or interval level of measurement. Ordinal measurement shows relative rankings whereby the intervals between numbers on the scale are not necessarily equal. At the interval level of measurement, distances between the numbers are equal. In both ordinal and interval measurement, there is no absolute zero point. Generally, interval level data permits more sophisticated statistical analyses (parametric statistics vs. nonparametric statistics); however, within the social sciences, there is much controversy about classification of the level of measurement and the appropriateness of selected statistical analyses (Knapp, 1990, 1993; LoBiondo-Wood &

Haber, 1998). Individual consideration and the acknowledgment of study limitations are the recommended actions (Knapp, 1990, 1993).

Typically, self-efficacy studies have reported means and standard deviations (Bandura, 1989; Lee & Bobko, 1994). The mean is a measure of central tendency, and the standard deviation is a measure of variability associated with interval level data; however, when reported with ordinal level data, limitations in interpretation must be acknowledged. When interpreting data, one must be aware that individuals who select a "3" response on a 10-point self-efficacy rating scale are not necessarily half as confident as individuals who select a "6" response. What can be interpreted is that the former individuals are less confident than the latter group as measured by that particular rating scale. Similarly, an individual with a mean subscale score of 7.0 is not exactly "twice" as confident as an individual scoring a mean of 3.5.

The best approach may be to adhere to the conventional analyses used in self-efficacy studies (interval level), interpret findings cautiously by acknowledging study limitations, repeat studies and compare results, and observe other outcome measures to substantiate findings. Because it is impossible to measure self-efficacy at such an exact level that distinguishes self-efficacy perceptions equally between individuals and between questionnaire response choices, researchers must go beyond this limitation to appreciate and value the findings generated in self-efficacy studies. Striving to control for other possible extraneous variables through a well-planned research design will enhance the validity and generalizability of findings (Ferguson, 2004).

Pretest Before Educational Intervention

When evaluating the effectiveness or impact of a specific educational intervention, the comparison of baseline data with outcome data strengthens the study. Using a pretest and posttest approach with a longitudinal sample will enhance the interpretability of findings. Administration of a self-efficacy measurement tool (e.g., the TSET) prior to the initiation of any specific transcultural teaching intervention, followed by a posttest administration immediately after the intervention, will permit the most control and decrease the risk of extraneous variables affecting results. Without a pretest, the researcher/educator cannot be sure that the educational intervention caused any change in the targeted population. Because it will be difficult to evaluate changes in cultural competency in the clinical area (see chapter 2), it will be increasingly important to evaluate changes in TSE. According to Bandura (1986, 1997), changes in self-efficacy through the use of pretest and posttest become more important to measure, especially when other performance outcome indicators may be difficult to evaluate.

The underlying premise is that self-efficacy is a mediator and predictor of outcome performance behaviors and outcomes (Bandura, 1996a, 1996b, 1997; Bandura & Schunk, 1981; Lent et al., 1993; Mone et al., 1995; Saks, 1995; Schunk, 1995).

Observe for Curricular/Program Consistency

Consistency in educational experiences between time of pretest and posttest is especially important when evaluating the impact of a curriculum or workshop series using an integrated approach to cultural competence development. The premise underlying a series of educational experiences (e.g., in a curriculum or clinical agency workshop series) is that each educational experience will build on previous learning. Learning experiences carefully coordinated to complement each other by weaving together learning in the cognitive, practical, and affective domains are most desirable. Active learning experiences designed to build on previous learning adds to depth and synthesis. Learners who are passive tourists, spectators, or mentally inattentive will not be actively engaged in the process of becoming culturally competent.

To accomplish the learning of cultural competence at higher depth and synthesis, careful thought and consideration must take into account the feasibility of offering sequenced, high-quality, learner-centered experiences. Sequencing courses, requiring prerequisites and corequisites that make sense conceptually, and avoiding class waivers simply for pure convenience will optimize the learning experience and help control for extraneous variables. Ideally, educators who want to measure the impact of transcultural nursing integrated throughout a curriculum (series of courses or educational experiences) should administer a pretest to all students similarly on their first class session of the first foundational transcultural nursing course and before exposure to transcultural educational interventions.

If some students are waived from taking the first foundational transcultural course to take several other courses first because of scheduling or other noneducational requests, the evaluation of TSE will be confounded by curricular inconsistency and by the weakening of transcultural concepts throughout. One desired outcome supporting sequencing of courses is that all students will have had the same exposure to transcultural concepts, skills, and theory. More enlightened learners within a class can reach higher levels of cultural competence development by sharing insights with each other at a higher level of synthesis. Learners without a common foundational experience will not have this advantage. Course expectations with mixed learner groups will have different, less effective educational outcomes because learning must be adjusted to accommodate learners without the prerequisite knowledge, skills, and values.

Determine Sufficient Sample Size

Determining sufficient sample size is a necessary precursor to enhance success in any study. Sample size will be determined by study purpose, literature review, conceptual framework, design, hypotheses/research questions, sampling technique, data collection, instruments, and data analyses. Although various sampling techniques may be employed, the advantages and disadvantages of different sampling techniques are not discussed here; rather, the focus is on sample size. However, it must be mentioned that most self-efficacy studies (and nursing studies) use nonprobability samples (convenience, purposive, quota).

First, all steps of the research process must be carefully considered before attempting to determine sample size. (The word "determine" is used rather than "calculate" because factors other than a mathematical formula must be considered.) Second, feasibility of attaining desired sample size must be appraised. Third, aiming for more than the minimum number in the sample is advisable because unforeseen circumstances may reduce the usable data (e.g., incomplete questionnaires and/or lack of identifiers for matching questionnaires).

The most common pitfall concerning sample size is that sample size is too small to provide robust data. Certain statistical analyses cannot even be performed via computerized statistical software packages unless a minimum number of cases are present. Occasionally, the statistical tests with small samples may be processed; however, statistical significance will never be achieved. The danger is that even if there is a change in the anticipated direction, it may not be detected in small sample sizes. Cohen's (1977) power analysis is a statistical procedure used to determine three levels of effect size for the desired power based on the probability of a type II error. (A type II error refers to the acceptance of a null hypothesis when it should have been rejected.) Statistical consultation and power analysis prior to the study implementation is valuable; however, other factors must be considered. Other considerations in sample size determination particularly relevant for proposed purposes in TSE studies are listed:

- Longitudinal studies require larger samples because mortality (drop outs) may occur.
- Longer time intervals between longitudinal data collection times require larger samples.
- Sample means will be affected by extreme scores, especially in small samples.

- Factor analysis studies require extremely large samples.
- Comparisons based on select demographic variables require sufficient respondents representing each demographic variable.

Collect Sufficient Demographic Data

The collection of sufficient demographic data will be valuable for four main reasons. First, demographic data will help determine whether the actual sample is truly representative of the targeted sample. Second, demographic data can be used to compare and contrast TSE perceptions between samples, permitting the expansion of scientific knowledge. Third, demographic data can be used to examine within-group differences based on demographic factors. Fourth, demographic data can help substantiate the underlying assumptions and directional conceptual relationships proposed in the CCC model and TSE Pathway.

Significant differences in TSE perceptions based on demographic variables can be desirable if differences are consistent with the underlying theoretical framework. For example, the CCC model purports that novice learners will have lower self-efficacy perceptions than advanced learners. Demographic data distinguishing between novices and advanced learners must therefore be collected and analyzed. In contrast, lack of statistically significant differences in TSE perceptions based on such variables as race, ethnicity, language, religion, or socioeconomic status supports the underlying theoretical assumption that all learners (despite race, ethnicity, etc.) benefit from transcultural nursing educational experiences to provide culturally congruent care for culturally different clients (Jeffreys & Smodlaka, 1998, 1999a, 1999b; Lim et al., 2004).

Deciding what type of demographic data should be collected will depend on the purpose and nature of the research investigation. It behooves the researcher/educator to critically appraise what demographic data could prove valuable prior to finalizing the study design and long before collecting data. Appendices G and H provide some examples. One general guideline is that sociodemographic questions should be placed last (Sudman & Bradburn, 1991). Some additional guidelines are listed:

- Demographic data that are never collected are lost forever. (Plan ahead.)
- Too many questions are overwhelming. (Ponder pertinence.)
- Unclear questions are confusing. (Make categories and questions clear.)
- Unnecessary personal questions are offensive. (Ask only what is necessary.)

- Avoid haphazard sequencing of questions. (Present the least non-threatening questions first, followed by more sensitive or personal questions [Sudman & Bradburn, 1991].)
- Data collected inconsistently have limited validity and usefulness. (Collect consistently.)
- The collection of invalid data is wasteful. (Collect carefully.)

Obtain Institutional Review Board Approval

Educators and/or researchers should be familiar with their institution's procedure and guidelines concerning Institutional Review Board (IRB) approval. Generally, teaching interventions and strategies for evaluating the effectiveness of teaching interventions does not require IRB approval if such teaching and outcome evaluations are typical expectations of the academic process and if findings will not be disseminated publicly. Initially, educators may not intend to publish, display, or present information; therefore, they do not seek IRB approval before beginning their assessments, interventions, and outcome evaluation. Unfortunately, this limits the usability of findings beyond the immediate institutional setting. The revitalization of nursing education must begin with educators taking active responsibility for using evidenced-based teaching interventions and sharing their knowledge with others through the dissemination of educational research (Diekelmann, 2002; Diekelmann & Ironside, 2002; Drevdahl, Stackman, Purdy, & Louie, 2002; Jeffreys, 2004; National League for Nursing, 2002a, 2002b; Riley, Beal, Levi, & McCausland, 2002; Storch & Gamroth, 2002; Tanner, 2002; Young & Diekelmann, 2002). Because IRB approval must be obtained before a study is initiated and because every educational intervention has the potential to make a difference (positive or negative) in the process of cultural competence development, educators must seriously consider the benefits and take the extra step in obtaining IRB approval.

Minimize Social Desirability Response Bias

Social desirability response bias refers to the tendency of some respondents to provide the "socially expected" response rather than true feelings (LoBiondo-Wood & Haber, 1998; Polit & Beck, 2004; Waltz, Strickland, & Lenz, 2005). Within the nursing profession, it could be assumed that cultural competence is a professional expectation; therefore, some researchers may be concerned about using self-report measurement tools to assess cultural competence. Bandura (1982) suggested that self-efficacy appraisals tend to be more conservative, especially when judgments are reported publicly, identification of respondents is possible, or direct observations of performance behaviors will occur. In other words, it may be "socially desirable" to present more conservative views of oneself. "Because there is no way to tell whether the respondent is telling the truth or responding in a socially desirable way, the researcher usually is forced to assume that the respondent is telling the truth" (LoBiondo-Wood & Haber, 1998, p. 318).

Although researchers must acknowledge that social desirability response bias may always exist in self-report instruments, several strategies may greatly reduce the effect of social desirability response bias on the results. To minimize social desirability response bias on the TSET, the author composed a letter of consent, informing respondents of the nature of the study, its educational benefits to nursing students, confidentiality, and voluntary participation (Jeffreys & Smodlaka, 1996). Several studies revealed that TSE perceptions were similar regardless of whether respondents replied anonymously. Anonymous data and matched data resulted in respondents selecting responses ranging from 1 (not confident) to 10 (totally confident) (Jeffreys & Smodlaka, 1996, 1998, 1999a, 1999b). Taking extra measures to assure student confidentiality and publicizing these measures can also minimize social desirability response bias. For example, asking respondents to wait to begin questionnaire completion until the data collector and instructor leave the room, appealing to respondents to complete questionnaires quietly and independently of each other, requesting students to place questionnaires in a sealed envelope, using barcodes for matching questionnaires, and reinforcing steps mentioned in the consent form can reassure respondents. The latter steps speak to the need for consistency in data collection.

Control Data Collection Procedures

Multiple data collectors and/or multiple data collection sites can complicate data collection consistency; however, steps can be taken to control data collection procedures. Collaboration with a liaison from each data collection site via written and telephone or personal correspondence should emphasize the need for consistent data collection procedures and clearly delineate the procedure steps. An information packet should contain a cover letter describing the nature of the study, instructions for instrument administration and return, and the instrument (and optical scanning sheets, if needed). Numbered steps and written statements for data collectors to read to respondents at specific intervals enhance consistency in data collection. A group setting with a designated time for instrument completion is the preferred method for collecting TSE data. Self-efficacy appraisal involves a complex thinking process that should be focused, undisturbed, uninterrupted, and precise. Eliminating distracters or other extraneous factors during instrument completion is vital for maximizing the validity of study results. If questionnaires are mailed to individuals, there is less control (consistency) in the data collection process. An accompanying letter should request individuals to set aside a specified amount of undisturbed time for instrument completion.

Watch for History as a Threat to Internal Validity

In addition to the independent variable, an event outside a study may occur that could influence the dependent variable. This threat to internal validity is referred to as history. Although researchers should be cognizant of various threats to internal validity (maturation, testing, instrumentation, mortality, and selection bias), only history will be highlighted here in relation to TSE and cultural competence development. Historical events could potentially influence perceptions positively or negatively. During longitudinal studies designed for the purpose of assessing the effectiveness of specific educational experiences for cultural competence development, researchers must closely watch for the possibility of outside influences. In a study involving one-time data collection, history as a threat to internal validity has a different impact. Noting any significant historical events immediately before data collection will be important, especially if comparison between samples at different points in time and/or geographic locations will be conducted. Watching for extraneous events and considering possible implications is an ongoing process. Several examples are provided:

- The JCAHO introduces "cultural competence" as a requirement for accreditation.
- A registered nurse licensing exam features new test items that target cultural competence.
- A health center receives grant funding to provide emergency care to new refugees from a foreign country.
- Following a local outbreak of tuberculosis, an emergency room is overcrowded with uninsured illegal immigrants seeking health care.
- A heroic act by a member of an ethnic and religious minority group is well publicized locally in a predominantly white Protestant community.
- Several racial riots break out on campus, seriously injuring several nursing students.
- Worldwide terrorist acts lead to war.
- National financial incentives emphasize the development of culture-specific health care.

Test Technology

A trial test run with the technology required to scan questionnaires, process data, and analyze data will prevent potential pitfalls from interfering with data use and interpretation. The technology trial test may require the expertise of computer experts, statisticians, psychometricians, and/or research assistants; therefore, early collaboration (before data collection) is essential. Various software programs are available for creating questionnaires; however, some programs may be more compatible with existing technological resources than others. It would be quite unfortunate if completed questionnaires cannot be scanned due to a technological problem. For example, the TSET formatted using Remark software must be scanned using Remark software; data can then easily be transferred into the SPSS program for data analysis. In contrast, the TSET typed format uses separate optical scanning forms. The completed optical scanning forms are then scanned using compatible software and an optical scanning machine. A computer expert may need to create a program for "reading" the scanning forms.

Without exploring the existing technological capabilities and/or limitations, a researcher may be stuck with data that cannot be easily processed. Checking the conditions of site licensing guidelines and/or the need for licensing renewals is another consideration. Computer technology and optical scanning equipment can ease the accuracy and speed at which questionnaires are processed. Testing technology in advance will avoid serious pitfalls.

KEY POINT SUMMARY

- Theoretical background information must be carefully considered when interpreting findings.
- Differentiating between individuals who demonstrate strong (resilient) self-efficacy, low self-efficacy (inefficacious), or supremely high self-efficacy (overconfidence) is integral to the interpretive process.
- It is presumed that individuals with resilient self-efficacy are highly motivated and actively seek help to maximize their transcultural nursing skills and cultural competence development. Resilient individuals would be the most likely to persist in cultural competence development and the most likely to achieve culturally congruent care actions.
- Low self-efficacy can affect cultural competence development directly, if individuals quit without even trying and then avoid

cultural assessments, or indirectly, through poor nursing outcomes and/or through negative psychological outcomes.

- Supremely efficacious individuals may be totally unaware of their weaknesses, underestimate the task or its importance, overlook the task, overestimate their abilities, and overrate their strengths. Overly confident individuals may not see the need for adequate preparation, restructuring of priorities, or time management to accommodate transcultural tasks.
- Although the identification of at-risk individuals followed by teaching interventions is one proposed purpose of interpreting self-efficacy perceptions, interpretation may also be conducted to guide curricular innovations.
- Strategies for avoiding pitfalls in TSE research design and interpretation include
  - Recognize limitations related to measurement level.
  - Pretest before educational intervention.
  - Observe for curricular/program consistency.
  - Determine sufficient sample size.
  - Collect sufficient demographic data.
  - Obtain IRB approval.
  - Minimize social desirability response bias.
  - Control data collection procedures.
  - Watch for history as a threat to internal validity.
  - Test technology.

Box 4.1   Educator-in-Action Vignette

Without adequate preparation and thoughtful consideration before and during research design, implementation, and data analysis, the interpretation of findings can be inaccurate and have devastating consequences. Consider the possible adverse effects of the following incorrect interpretations. Contrast the potential effects of the alternative, improved interpretation.

Situation A

Using the TSET pretest and posttest results from a sample of 15 senior baccalaureate nursing students who enrolled in a transcultural nursing course elective, t test results indicate statistically insignificant changes in TSE on all subscales.

Professor Quick states, "These results prove that the transcultural nursing course elective is not significant in developing cultural competence. We should cancel this course and reallocate funds toward the medical-surgical clinical courses."

Professor Best states, "It is not surprising that statistically significant results did not occur with such a small, self-selected convenience sample. The transcultural nursing course should be a required prerequisite or corequisite course to the clinical courses to enhance cultural competence development and permit application. A larger, more representative, and diverse (not self-selected) sample will decrease the probability of a type II error."

Situation B

The following TSET scores are obtained:

	Sample Mean (n = 87)	Standard Deviation	Case 1	Case 2	Case 3	Case 4
Cognitive	5.43	2.21	5.86	9.22	3.07	6.54
Practical	6.34	1.96	6.97	9.34	4.27	6.97
Affective	7.56	1.74	8.04	9.87	5.71	7.66

Professor Quick states, "Cognitive subscale scores show that Case 2 is more than three times as knowledgeable about culture-specific care as Case 3. It would be a good idea to match Cases 2 and 3 together because Case 2 would be a good role model. Cognitive subscale scores are lowest overall, so it will be more important to emphasize knowledge (content) about specific cultures. Affective subscale scores are highest, so this dimension of learning should not be a priority. The curriculum should be modified based on these results."

Professor Best states, "Consistent with the underlying conceptual framework of the CCC model, the data suggest that students in this sample are least confident about their knowledge and most confident about their attitudes, values, and beliefs. Learning that purposely integrates cognitive, practical, and affective dimensions optimizes learning outcomes; therefore, educational interventions should continue to emphasize and integrate all three components. Besides, affective learning is viewed as the most powerful in influencing professional development and cognitive learning."

Scores for Case 2 suggest that he or she may be overly confident, whereas scores for Case 3 suggest that he or she may be inefficacious. According to the CCC model and the TSE Pathway, both Case 2 and Case 3 could be identified as "at risk" for providing culturally incongruent care; however, limitations due to measurement prevent absolute categorization or exact comparisons of scores between individuals. Follow-up assessment and intervention with the identified at-risk individuals is appropriate and indicated. We should not generalize these first-time results and change the curriculum, but rather we should continue to collect data and compare results."

PART II

Educational Activities for Easy Application

CHAPTER 5

Academic Settings

Any educational setting can provide numerous, ongoing opportunities for promoting cultural competence; however, the academic setting has the potential to make the greatest impact. Primarily, this is true because the main function of the academic setting is "education" and the primary student role is "learning." Learning can be maximized through a well-planned, coordinated approach (see Figure 5.1). Leininger (1995b) proposed four approaches for effectively integrating transcultural nursing within the academic setting: (a) transcultural concepts, skills, and principles integrated within an existing curriculum; (b) select culture care modules incorporated within a curriculum; (c) a series of coordinated, substantive transcultural nursing courses with field experiences; and (d) a major degree program or track in transcultural nursing (graduate level).

The first approach is emphasized in this chapter because it has the broadest and most immediate application across various academic settings and degree programs. In addition, the integrated approach has the potential to positively affect the greatest number of "future" nurses. Without an initial, formalized exposure to transcultural nursing, how will nursing students even know of its existence, realize its significance, and develop the beginning knowledge, skills, values, and confidence necessary for learning and performing culturally congruent nursing care? Furthermore, how will students be aware of the vast possibilities for ongoing learning in cultural competence development or advanced degree options? Early, stimulated interest in transcultural nursing may later lead to a desire to pursue a specialized degree program or track in transcultural nursing.

Lifelong, ongoing cultural competence development is an essential professional expectation presently and in the future; therefore, it becomes extremely urgent that initial education emphasizes cultural competence. Entry-level education offers the greatest possibilities, particularly the first nursing "fundamentals" course, because it provides the foundation for

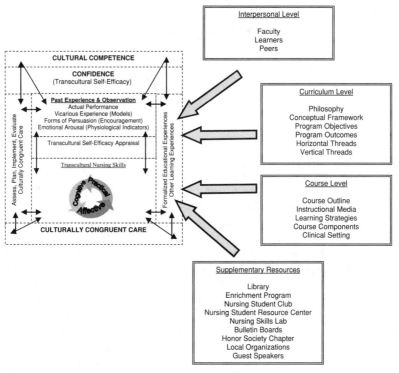

Figure 5.1 Academic settings.

all future nursing courses and nursing practice. Optimally, a required pre-requisite or corequisite transcultural nursing course will further enhance the possibility for a stronger foundation for cultural competence development; however, an additional course may not be feasible, especially with the time and credit constraints of associate degree nursing programs. Numerically, entry-level education has the potential to make enormous strides in cultural competence development because enrollment in such programs is greater than any other degree programs. This educational and professional goal can only occur with well-qualified, committed nursing faculty and through the use of culturally congruent teaching–learning strategies that address students' diverse cultural values and beliefs (CVB).

Nurse educators are empowered to make a tremendous difference by introducing, fostering, and nurturing cultural competence development. Each individual faculty member is empowered to make a positive difference; however, the greatest impact will be achieved through a coordinated, holistic group effort that thoughtfully weaves together nursing course components, nursing curriculum, and supplementary resources. Certain factors within the academic setting may support cultural competence development, yet other factors may restrict its development.

This chapter aims to (a) uncover, discover, and explore educational opportunities (within academia) for promoting cultural competency; (b) describe action-focused strategies for educational innovation; and (c) present ideas for evaluation (and re-evaluation) of educational innovation implementation. Figures, tables, "Innovations in Cultural Competence Education" boxes, and the "Educator-in-Action" vignette provide supplementary information to expand on narrative text features. Major emphasis is placed on individual instructor appraisal and course-level appraisal.

FACULTY SELF-ASSESSMENT

Promoting cultural competency in academia requires considerable, sincere effort that must begin with self-assessment. Self-assessment is a process in which the nurse educator systematically appraises the various dimensions that can impact the educational process and the achievement of educational outcomes (Jeffreys, 2004). A systematic assessment can be initiated using the cultural dimensions listed in Table 1.2 and illustrated in Figure 5.2. The realization that there are multidimensional variables influencing student–faculty interaction is overwhelming; yet, these variables are essential to evaluate before developing a culturally congruent educational approach. Sometimes nurse educators may be "unconsciously incompetent" in their educational approach with culturally diverse (different) students. According to Purnell (2003), one is unconsciously incompetent when one is not aware of cultural differences or when one unknowingly carries out actions that are not culturally congruent. Behaviors such as cultural blindness, cultural imposition, and culturally incongruent actions can cause cultural pain to others (Leininger & McFarland, 2002). Consciously attempting to implement culturally congruent behaviors and avoiding incompetence is a key component in facilitating cultural competence development among culturally diverse learners.

First, self-awareness of one's own CVB is essential. Although the nursing faculty member may be immersed within the "culture" of nursing education and be familiar with long-held nursing education CVB, it is important to be aware of the unconscious and conscious CVB that exist in nursing education and in one's own values and belief systems. Faculty must be aware that their own CVB, held long before entering into the

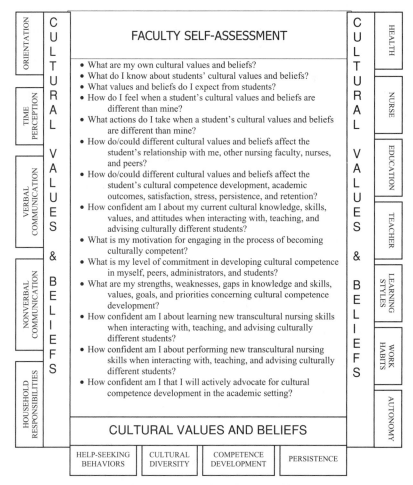

Figure 5.2 Faculty self-assessment. Adapted from Jeffreys, M. R. (2004). *Nursing student retention: Understanding the process and making a difference.* New York, Springer Publishing, 169. Used by permission, Springer Publishing Company, Inc., New York 10036.

nursing culture, may influence values, beliefs, practices, behaviors, and actions consciously and unconsciously. For example, a nursing faculty member whose traditional cultural values favor direct eye contact for all communication and view lack of eye contact suspiciously will need to be consciously aware of his or her underlying values and beliefs and aim to consciously avoid distrusting students based solely on this nonverbal cue (Jeffreys, 2004).

Second, awareness of one's knowledge about different CVB, especially the CVB that most directly affect the teaching–learning process and cultural competence development, must be explored (see Figure 5.2). Although Table 1.2 presents a snapshot approach of selected CVB that may impact the educational experience, it does allow for a quick comparison of different CVB. One benefit of this approach is that it evokes the awareness that there may be other CVB in various cultures of which the nurse educator is unaware. The realization that one is not and cannot always be "culturally competent" is often a powerful awakening. Becoming conscious of one's incompetence is often a humbling experience that often sparks a desire for obtaining cultural knowledge. Awareness of differences and similarities between values and beliefs espoused in higher education, nursing education, and individual student CVB can also lend new insight into why conflicts, misunderstandings, and alternate priorities predominate. Such raised awareness can help determine whether specific factors are supportive or restrictive toward the goal of developing cultural competence among culturally diverse students that can guide cultural-specific educational interventions.

Embedded in this self-assessment is the appraisal of one's understanding about the multidimensional factors influencing nursing student learning, achievement, retention, success, and cultural competence development. Educational views, policy, learning styles, and values about education differ across cultures (Callister, Khalaf, & Keller, 2000; Crow, 1993; Keane, 1993; Nurmi & Aunola, 2001; Purnell & Paulanka, 2003; Rew, 1996; Stigler & Hiebert, 1998; Winters & Owens, 1993; Yoder, 2001) and impact learning, achievement, and persistence (Labun, 2002; Nurmi & Aunola, 2001; Ransdell, 2001a, 2001b; Ransdell, Hawkins, & Adams, 2001a, 2001b; Yoder, 1996). Unless nurse educators conduct a systematic appraisal of all multidimensional components, full understanding will not truly be achieved. Nurse educators should reflect on the last time a thorough, updated review of the literature on cultural competence, the teaching–learning process, and culturally diverse students was conducted. Appraisal of one's desire for updated knowledge and commitment should be critically determined. Evaluating one's knowledge about student expectations and perceptions should be appraised. Lack of knowledge or limited knowledge in this area identifies areas for further self-development; however, one must have the desire to obtain knowledge and be committed to the pursuit of such an endeavor or knowledge quest. Finally, self-assessment should conclude with a listing of strengths, weaknesses, gaps in knowledge, goals, commitment, and priorities.

The nurse educator must assess one's cultural desire or motivation for engaging in the process of becoming culturally competent. Within this construct of cultural desire is the concept of caring for others

(Campinha-Bacote, 2003). Cultural knowledge is the process of searching and obtaining a thorough educational foundation about various CVB in an attempt to comprehend and empathize with others' perspectives. Along with awareness, cultural desire and cultural knowledge are essential steps toward becoming culturally competent (Campinha-Bacote, 2003). Thoroughly reflecting on the feelings experienced and actions taken when student's CVB are different from one's own CVB can further one's insight. Because the process of cultural competence is ongoing, the nurse educator should examine one's commitment toward achieving this goal. True commitment necessitates time, energy, persistence, extra effort to overcome obstacles, and willingness to learn from mistakes.

Comprehensive understanding, skill, and desire are essential but not enough to effectively make a positive difference in cultural competence development. The author believes that resilient transcultural self-efficacy (TSE) (confidence) is the integral component necessary in the process of cultural competence development (of self and in others). TSE is the mediating factor that enhances persistence in cultural competence development, despite obstacles, hardships, or stressors. Resilient TSE perceptions embrace lifelong learning in the quest to become "more" culturally competent and in the quest to assist others (learners) to become more culturally competent. Educators with resilient TSE perceptions persist in their endeavors to be active transcultural advocates or promoters of cultural competence in all dimensions of the educational setting and professional practice.

Faculty self-assessment as "active promoter of cultural competence development" is a necessary precursor for successful strategy development. Table 5.1 provides a guide for appraising values, beliefs, and actions and for determining whether one is an active role model in cultural competence development. It is proposed that the "actions taken to promote cultural competence development" is what makes one an active role model. Table 5.1 can also provide a guide for organizational self-assessment to determine if schools of nursing, educational institutions, and organizations are "active promoters" or if there are factors restricting cultural competence development.

Participation in cultural competence conferences, workshops, events, meetings, and relevant professional memberships exemplify a professional commitment to lifelong learning and cultural competence development that can be motivating and uplifting to students. Professional nurses serve as role models through their commitment to learning and the nursing profession. Because students have most exposure to the nursing profession through faculty guidance, nurse educators exert powerful influence on students. If faculty do not value cultural competence educational activities for their own professional development, then it is hard to imagine

Table 5.1 Nurse Educator's Self-Assessment: Active Promoter of Cultural
Competence Development

Promoter	Values, beliefs, and actions	Promoter
Yes	Views cultural competence as important in own life *and shares beliefs with students*[a]	No
Yes	Views cultural competence as important in students' education, professional development, and future practice *and shares view with students*	No
Yes	Views own nurse educator role to include active involvement in promoting cultural competence development among students *and shares view with students*	No
Yes	Routinely updates own knowledge and skills to enhance cultural competence *and shares relevant information with students*	No
Yes	Attends professional events concerning cultural competence development *and shares positive and relevant experiences with students*	No
Yes	Views professional event participation concerning cultural competence development as important in students' education and/or professional development and future practice *and shares view with students*	No
Yes	*Offers incentives to encourage student participation in professional events focused on cultural competence*	No
Yes	Maintains professional partnerships focused on cultural competence development *and shares positive and relevant experiences with students*	No
Yes	Maintains membership(s) in professional organizations whose primary mission is cultural competence development *and shares positive and relevant experiences with students*	No
Yes	Views student memberships in nursing organizations/associations (whose primary mission is cultural competence development) as important in students' education and/or professional development, and future practice *and shares view with students*	No
Yes	*Offers incentives to encourage student participation in memberships in nursing organizations/associations committed to cultural competence development*	No
Yes	Recognizes actual and potential barriers hindering student's development of cultural competence *and initiates strategies to remove barriers*	No
Yes	*Implements strategies to encourage student development of cultural competence*	No
Yes	*Evaluates strategies implemented to encourage student development cultural competence*	No

[a] Active promoter/facilitator actions are indicated by *italics*.
Adapted from Jeffreys, M. R. (2004). *Nursing student retention: Understanding the process and making a difference*. New York, Springer. Used by permission, Springer Publishing Company, Inc., New York 10036.

that they would have a positive impact on encouraging students' active development. Similarly, if nurse educators are actively involved in cultural competence activities, yet do not actively publicize their views, involvement, participation, and contribution, positive professional role modeling will not be evident to students. Vicarious learning through role modeling and forms of persuasion (encouragement) are powerful influences on self-efficacy appraisal, motivation, and persistence behaviors (Bandura, 1986).

After self-assessment, nurse educators who have not optimally shared positive views, values, beliefs, and experiences with students should make a concerted effort to do so. It is, however, not enough to profess values and beliefs to students; nurse educators must be sincerely committed and take positive actions to "make a difference" and enhance cultural competence development. To do this, nurse educators must recognize actual and potential barriers hindering student's cultural competence development, propose innovative solutions, take action, initiate strategies, evaluate educational innovations, and create new innovations based on evaluative data.

EVALUATION IN THE ACADEMIC SETTING

As students, educators, administrators, and health care consumers become more astute collectively in recognizing that culturally congruent health care is a right—not a privilege—it becomes increasingly urgent to closely examine how visible (or invisible) cultural competency development is in the academic setting. At the undergraduate and graduate setting, examination at the curricular, program, school, and course level requires courage, commitment, time, energy, and a systematic plan. A systematic evaluative inquiry can be guided by two additional questions: (a) To what degree is cultural competence an integral component? and (b) How do all the cultural components fit together? (see Figure 5.3). A thorough evaluation serves as a valuable precursor to informed decisions, responsible actions, and new diagnostic-prescriptive educational innovations. The following sections address key features for inquiry, action, and innovation within the academic setting.

Curriculum

Systematic curriculum evaluation via quantitative and qualitative methods helps identify program strengths, weaknesses, inconsistencies, and gaps. Reflective self-appraisal on an individual level and a program level is necessary for enhancing the scholarship of teaching (Drevdahl, Stackman, Purdy, & Louie, 2002; Young & Diekelmann, 2002). Concept mapping that focuses on cultural competence as a concept helps trace the concept

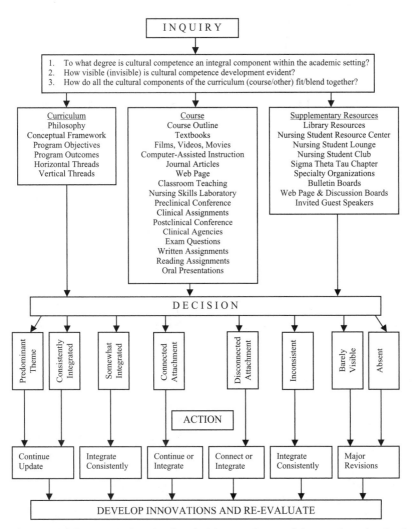

Figure 5.3 Systematic inquiry for decision, action, and innovation: Academic setting.

throughout the curriculum. On close scrutiny, curricular threads of culture and cultural competency should be equally and substantially evident throughout the program's philosophy, conceptual framework, program objectives, program outcomes, courses, and all course components. Examination of curricular threads must differentiate between horizontal and vertical threads. For example, horizontal threads are interested in the "process" of learning; therefore, horizontal threads must be introduced early, integrated purposely, and intricately woven throughout the curriculum to create a durable fabric that provides long-lasting learning and desirable outcomes.

In contrast, vertical threads are "content" oriented; they build from simple foundational content to more complex content. For example, moving from nursing care of the individual to family and then community demonstrates movement from simple dimensions to more complex dimensions. Applying "content" to care of the individual, care of the family, and care of the community should consider cultural-specific measures within the plan of care. For example, the "content" of breast cancer screening should address culturally congruent measures to optimize screening by reaching out to culturally diverse individuals, families, and communities. Curricular vertical and horizontal threads should be complementary, consistent, and appropriate for each educational level. Appropriate selection and sequencing of courses should be justified with clear rationale. Foundational prerequisite courses, corequisite courses, and subsequent courses must fit together and build on each other.

Although less discussed in the nursing literature, strategy mapping throughout the curriculum is another important evaluative method. Strategy mapping traces various student-centered learning approaches, thereby assessing another necessary curricular dimension. Because diverse learners have diverse learning needs, strengths, values, and beliefs, weaving different multidimensional active learning activities throughout the course and curriculum will be most beneficial (Brookfield, 1986; Gaffney, 2000; Kelly, 1997; Williams & Calvillo, 2002; Yoder, 2001). Students' CVB will influence how various strategies are valued, interpreted, and used; therefore, nurse educators should take this into consideration while planning, implementing, and evaluating activities. Students need to understand and appreciate the conditions under which specific learning strategies may be more or less effective rather than assuming that certain ones are best (Pintrich & Garcia, 1994). Explaining the value of different teaching–learning activities may be indicated to optimally facilitate learning among culturally diverse and academically diverse learners.

Specific activities have advantages and disadvantages. Pairing students eliminates the potential for an audience and enhances the potential for in-depth quality student interactions that can foster cognitive and affective growth (Christiaens & Baldwin, 2002). Groups, however, provide greater opportunities for diverse thinking. Outcome benefits can be maximized with clear directions, group rules, well-matched group composition, effective leadership, immediate feedback and guidance, reflection, and adequate time allocation (Huff, 1997). Story-telling with reflection is another effective strategy, especially among culturally diverse learners (Koenig & Zorn, 2002). For many students, gaming, debates, and role play provide an effective mechanism for active, fun learning that results in cognitive, psychomotor, and/or affective outcomes (Candela, Michael, & Mitchell, 2003; Cowen & Tesh, 2002; Jeffreys, 1991; Kramer, 1995; Pimple, Schmidt, & Tidwell, 2003); yet, individual competitiveness may be contrary to some students' CVB. Classroom lectures must be routinely appraised for diversity content (Scisney-Matlok, McCloud, & Barnard, 2001) and should be partnered with lively discussion and other interactive activities. The Internet (web-based courses) provides opportunities for interactive learning in pairs, small groups, and large groups via individual e-mail, group e-mails, course chat rooms, and course discussion boards (Bolan, 2003; Christianson, Tiene, & Luft, 2002; Harden, 2003; Koeckeritz, Malkiewicz, & Henderson, 2002; MacIntosh, MacKay, Mallet-Boucher, & Wiggins, 2002; Sternberger, 2002). Most recently, web casting permits audio and visual presentations via the Internet, including live class participation via personal computers (DiMaria-Ghalili, Ostrow, & Rodney, 2005; Ostrow & DiMaria-Ghalili, 2005). Students must be computer literate, confident, and motivated if computer-based strategies are to be effective. Nurse educators have many learner-centered student interactive strategies from which to choose; however, the educator must be adequately prepared, knowledgeable of student variables, committed, and caring if strategies are to be successful (Jeffreys, 2004).

Inconsistent and/or insufficient integration of cultural competence curricular threads, learning activities, strategies, opportunities, and incentives throughout the nursing curriculum restricts cultural competence development and is confusing to students. Curricular inconsistency is incongruent with the creation of a true community of culturally diverse nursing learners—essential for culturally inclusive professional socialization, development, and growth. Curricular inconsistency is also counterproductive to earlier cultural competence-promoting efforts; inconsistency confounds students and compounds educational outcomes. In contrast, consistent vertical and horizontal threads, purposely woven throughout the curriculum, are a program strength that can only support student learning and success.

Curricular mapping and a detailed critique of the philosophy, conceptual framework, program objectives, program outcomes, and curricular threads is an ambitious endeavor, requiring much courage, humility, honesty, and dedication. It is often a humbling experience to realize that one's curriculum necessitates an intensive overhaul or detailed tune-up in cultural competence (or any other area as well). Concept mapping and strategy mapping provide methods for tracing curricular threads and learning activities, identifying gaps, and detecting overlapping areas. More recently, electronic-based strategies have facilitated the ease of ongoing and collaborative curriculum evaluation (Miller, Koyanagi, & Morgan,

2005). Inquiries must extend beyond the immediate nursing program to examine the possibility of seamless articulation into more advanced nursing programs (that build on foundational cultural competence learning) at the same school, neighboring and/or affiliating schools, and/or nursing programs nationally recognized as leaders in cultural competence development.

Certain factors will enhance the ability to conduct an intensive curriculum critique. These include psychological factors, practical factors, and expertise factors. Ideally, all conditions should be favorable for a critique to be most successful and valid. Psychological factors include intrinsic motivation, extrinsic motivation, commitment, willingness to make changes, open-mindedness, satisfaction, minimal stress, workplace harmony, positive group dynamics, and perceived positive reinforcement. Practical factors include time, workload, financial resources, administrative support, secretarial support, technical resources, facilities, and energy. Expertise factors include the level of expertise (educational preparation and actual task experience) in evaluation, curriculum development and evaluation, curriculum process via group interaction, concept mapping, cultural competence development, teaching and learning cultural competence, teaching and learning process, adult learners, culturally diverse students, and learner characteristics.

Unfortunately, there is a critical shortage of nursing faculty that is projected to increase in the future (Adams, Murdock, Valiga, McGinnis, & Wolfertz, 2002; NLN, 2002a, 2002b; Rizzolo, 2002; Stevenson, 2003). Furthermore, the number of faculty formally prepared in the teaching and learning of nursing and in the curriculum development is tragically declining. For example, the number of graduates specifically prepared in nursing education via master's programs with education tracks has declined to only 116 graduates in 2000 (Rizzolo, 2002). In addition, the number of faculty formally prepared with courses in transcultural nursing is grossly inadequate (Andrews, 1995; Jeffreys, 2002; Leininger, 1995b). Combining the desired faculty attributes to include preparation in both areas results in even lower numbers. Faculty experienced in curriculum and cultural competency will need to lead and mentor others in this evaluative process.

Course

Close scrutiny at the course level (undergraduate and graduate) should assess whether cultural competency development is emphasized substantially, equally, and symmetrically in all dimensions and course components. This can begin by examining all components of the course outline: course description, course objectives, course topics, student-expected outcomes, learning activities, course assignments, and methods of evaluation. Using the general questions depicted in Figure 5.3, nurse educators can conduct a systematic inquiry, make a decision, choose an action, and then develop innovations. For example, if a nurse educator decides that "care of culturally diverse clients" mentioned in the course description is "barely visible" in the other course outline components, the action chosen should be to make major revisions, develop innovations, and re-evaluate within a specified time period. Collaboration with other faculty teaching in the nursing program and outside experts will be essential to the overall curricular goals and process. As a second example, a nurse educator may decide that the course topics present cultural competence as an "add-on" or "disconnected attachment." Thereafter, the chosen action will be to connect together, or better still, to integrate as a horizontal thread.

Inquiry at the course level also includes all instructional media (e.g., textbooks, films, videos, movies, computer-assisted instruction, journal articles, web page, PowerPoint), course components (e.g., classroom, nursing skills laboratory, clinical, and/or immersion experience), teaching–learning activities, and methods of evaluation (e.g., written assignments, presentations, exam questions). Each of the following sections highlights several select course-level components, providing examples of course-specific innovations. It is beyond the scope of this chapter to detail all elements. Readers are encouraged to critique the innovations presented, as well as to modify, adapt, and create new innovations for the teaching and learning of cultural competence.

Textbooks and Reading Assignments

Appraising textbooks carefully using preset criteria provides a systematic evaluation of textbook options (Schoolcraft & Novotny, 2000). Although evaluation of content areas, supplementary features, cost, date of publication, and usability are important considerations, nurse educators must consider other aspects, especially if the needs of academically diverse and culturally diverse students are to be met. Textbook selection must be guided by learner characteristics, type of course, intended purpose of reading assignments, textbook features, coordination with other course components, and connection with other courses (prerequisite, corequisite, and subsequent).

It is important to remember that it is not only the textbook that can make a difference in the learning process and the achievement of learning outcomes, but rather how the textbook is used (or not used). Accurate knowledge and comprehension about learner characteristics is a necessary precursor to textbook selection and the preparation of reading assignments. Box 5.1 presents an overview of learner characteristics

---

Box 5.1   Innovations in cultural competence education: Assessment
of learner characteristics

Type of Course
____Required __Elective ____AAS ___BS generic ___RN-BS __Masters __Doctorate
Prerequisites _____Corequisites _____
Transcultural __Clinical__Theory __Research __Issues __Leadership ___
Community __Other_____
Learner Characteristics
Age ____Adult learners ____Traditional age students Age range_____Average ___
Gender__Female__Male
Language____English as first language (EPL)____English as second (other) language
(ESL)
ESL Predominant Languages _____
Prior Educational Experience _____U.S. high school diploma_____Foreign HS
diploma____GED____General ____Academic__Honors ____Advanced placement
____Vocational
Remedial Education____Reading ____Writing ____Math ____Biology ___Chemistry
___Other
Prior College Experience ____Transfer credits, no degree____U.S. ___Foreign
____Community college ____Senior college ____Graduate school
____Associate degree ____Bachelor's degree __Masters' degree ___Doctorate
____Nursing degree ___Non-nursing degree
Enrollment History___Continuous___Course withdrawals__Stopouts
Enrollment Status_____Full-time _____Part-time_____Matriculated
____Nonmatriculated
Prior Health Care Experience_____Unlicensed health care personnel
____Licensed health care personnel ___LPN__RN__Other
Prior Work Experience ____None__Displaced homemaker__Second career
Employment Status ___Full-time ___Part-time___On-campus ___Off-campus
Financial Status ___Disadvantaged ___Financial aid__Subsidized loans _____
Work-study
Family Role Responsibilities _____Single parent _____Parent_____Spouse
___Caregiver _____Other
Group Disparity_____African American or black_____Hispanic _____Native
American
____underrepresented Asian _____other Asian ____White, disadvantaged ___White
Ethnic Diversity   Predominant student groups_____
    New immigrant student groups_____
    New refugee student groups_____
    Foreign student groups_____
    Other student groups_____
Religious Diversity Predominant student religions_____
    Other student religions_____
Institutional Characteristics
____Open enrollment_____Public_____Private, non-religious ____Religious
(type)_____Historically black college or university (HBCU)
____Hispanic-serving ____Tribal college____Community college ____Senior
college ____Graduate degree college_____Urban ____Suburban ___Rural
___Commuter__Residential

Nursing Program Characteristics
___Weekend program ____Evening program ___Day and evening program
___Cohort program___Cooperative-learning-work program___Distance learning
____Web-based___Web-enhanced

helpful in developing a profile of learner characteristics. For example, if many nursing students are financially challenged, it is unrealistic to expect that a supplementary textbook will be purchased to complete two required class readings. In fact, such expectations may cause undue stress to financially challenged students. A better approach may be to supplement one main textbook with select journal articles available online with full-text access or on reserve in the library. Several brief journal articles, featuring select cultural topics can be used to enhance cultural competence development by creatively integrating the articles with other course activities. Optional readings concerning culture (or any topic) send a mixed message to students. For example, students may perceive that cultural considerations in nursing care is "optional," rather than an expected, integral component in providing quality nursing care, and never complete the reading.

As another example, an academically diverse student group will need much guidance on how to become active readers, use tables and graphs effectively, analyze and synthesize material, formulate questions, and highlight important information (Mertig, 2003). A new student orientation or course orientation that customizes prereading strategies, time management, active reading strategies, note-taking, and study skills to the nursing course will be most beneficial in enhancing success. Without reinforced guidance, students may not see the importance of textbook case studies, research briefs, clinical snapshots, or other textbook chapter features concerning culturally diverse clients. As a result, students may neglect to read these sections. Consistent with trends in higher education, the numbers of academically diverse undergraduate nursing students, such as ESL students or students who completed remedial courses have also increased. Nurse educators can further assist diverse students by

- Selecting an easy-to-read, appropriate textbook that is enhanced with visual aids
- Identifying a reasonable number of reading assignments that students can complete
- Encouraging use of a dictionary to look up unfamiliar words
- Preparing advance organizers, discussion questions, or outlines to focus reading
- Developing study guides that correlate with course and reading assignments
- Organizing weekly study groups to discuss readings and answer questions

Examining the textbook for the age, gender, and cultural diversity of registered nurses depicted in illustrations, photos, or case exemplars is another important consideration to promote inclusion and foster cultural competence development. Identifying gaps between learner characteristics and textbook case studies provides the opportunity for nurse educators to supplement readings with other examples featuring cultures both similar and different from those of learners. Such supplements are valuable whether the course is an undergraduate medical–surgical nursing course, a required core course in the master's degree curriculum, or any other course on any degree level.

Films, Movies, or Videos

Films, movies, or videos provide unique opportunities to enhance student cognitive, psychomotor, and affective learning. For the purposes of this chapter, "films, movies, and videos" are referred to simply as "videos." Through videos, students are exposed to a combined audio and visual medium that can enhance learning, especially among visual learners. If used appropriately, videos can expose students to a wide variety of new situations and cultural groups in a short amount of time that ordinarily they may not have the opportunity to encounter at all or for some time. Unfortunately, videos also have the potential for perpetrating stereotypes unless students are properly guided.

The best learning can take place if students are appropriately guided toward what to focus on in the video. A set of guided objectives, expected outcomes, and/or preset discussion questions can direct student's attention toward achieving the desired learning outcomes. Pausing the video at strategic points is beneficial to maximize active learning (Ulrich & Glendon, 1999). For example, the nurse educator can elaborate on key components, ask probing questions to stimulate further inquiry, direct learners to reflect on the last segment viewed, and provide opportunity for guided class questions and/or discussion before proceeding on with film. Pauses permit self-reflection, class dialog, synthesis, clarification, and organized compartmentalization of learning "chunks" before proceeding to new learning. New questions or areas of guided focus can assist learners (especially novices) about what to look for, thereby serving as a jump-start for critical thinking about cultural competence.

Cautioning viewers about the dangers of stereotyping based on the scenarios depicted in the video recognizes limitations but permits a partial insight into a different, emic (insider's) view. An outsider from a different culture may gain a new viewpoint. Through organized class discussion, a student who is an "insider" into the depicted culture may also gain a new perspective on how outsiders (classmates) view certain CVB, while also being able to add his or her perspective on CVB presented in the video. Every video should be evaluated as to how it potentially perpetuates misperceptions, inaccuracies, and biases within nursing, health care, and particular cultural groups. The instructor is empowered to make a significant difference by developing cultural competence in students concerning every topic. Stopping the video to describe application to various cultural groups emphasizes the importance of culture and effectively links culture with other course components. When comparing and contrasting cultures, focused questions can assist students in recognizing subtle differences in various cultures (Ulrich & Glendon, 1999).

Whether videos viewed outside of class are required or supplemental can tremendously impact learning outcomes. For example, if a video on "Chinese healing" is supplemental rather than required, then the perception is that it is (a) unnecessary, (b) less important than "required" assignments, and/or (c) optional. Similarly, if a video is "required" but is not connected to the other course components, assignments, or discussions, it is really a disconnected attachment that needs to be connected or integrated effectively throughout the course (or ideally, the curriculum).

Educational course videos may focus on varied topics such as (a) general transcultural nursing principles, (b) a particular cultural group, (c) comparison between several cultural groups, (d) multidisciplinary health care, (e) clinical topics with cultural competence addressed, (f) clinical topics without cultural competence addressed, (g) client-centered teaching, or (h) conferences and meetings. Clinical topic videos should be critically appraised for relevance within and between cultural groups. For example, videos that include skin assessment should take into account differences based on physical appearance (e.g., variations in skin pigmentation, healing, and scar formation), cultural practices (e.g., tattoos, body piercing, male and female circumcision), cultural values (e.g., taboos, modesty in exposing skin to examiners of different genders, ages, cultures, and religions). Although the film may not address this, or may address these issues minimally, the nurse educator has the potential to make a difference by asking students to reflect on different client situations, asking questions, story-telling about actual clinical incidents, and presenting case studies (see Box 5.2).

Box 5.2   Innovations in cultural competence education: In-class video teaching–learning activities

1. Select videos that accurately depict culturally diverse clients, nurses, and other health care providers.
2. For all videos, but especially for clinically focused videos with little cultural diversity, note limitations and develop learning activities

(questions, reflection, discussion, role playing, story-telling) to expand on clinical focus by addressing cultural issues.

3. Create a guided set of objectives/learning outcomes that corresponds/links with (or expands on) other aspects of course content/objectives, videos, patient care assignments, reading assignments, specific for the video teaching–learning experience.

4. Include objectives and learning outcomes for video teaching–learning activity in course outline and/or class handout. (Discussion questions and prerequisite reading can provide necessary background information to facilitate achievement of desired learning outcomes.)

5. Review objectives and learning outcomes with students, emphasizing learner-centered feature aimed at developing cultural competence. Give students a guided "movie preview."

6. Prepare a set of guided questions, comments, alternate case scenario with different cultural dimensions within the same cultural group, alternate case scenario with different cultural dimensions among different cultural groups, and pause points for strategic points in the video. (Note that select questions and scenarios can also be divided among several small groups for a small-group discussion that is followed by a large-group discussion or debriefing session.)

7. Interject comments, questions, and invite student questions and comments.

8. Note areas of interested discussion, student questions and responses, weakness, strengths, and gaps.

9. Obtain students' verbal and/or written feedback concerning video teaching–learning activity.

10. Incorporate results from steps 8 and 9 into future course offerings and curricular revision.

Computer-Assisted Instruction

Preparing computer-literate graduates of nursing programs who exercise critical thinking, clinical decision making, and reflection is an absolute necessity now and in the future (Mueller, Pullen, & McGee, 2002). In particular, the future demands that nurses exercise critical thinking and clinical decision making that consider client's cultural values, beliefs, and practices. Empirical evidence supports that computer-assisted instruction (CAI) can enhance self-efficacy in clinical decision making, as well as create a link between theoretical and clinical learning without the fear of jeopardizing client safety (Madorin & Iwasiw, 1999; Mertig, 2003; Weis & Guyton-Simmons, 1998). Within the context of cultural competence education, this means that students can potentially interact with a wide sampling of clients who are culturally different than the student without fear of making cultural mistakes. Students may have guided practice without the instructor present (Boyce & Winne, 2000), thereby decreasing the anxiety of being observed, judged, or graded. Especially for adult learners who are self-directed and desire immediate feedback for performance, CAI offers a forum for independent learning, immediate feedback, clinical decision making, and critical thinking in a nonthreatening environment; transcultural self-efficacy (TSE) perceptions will be positively influenced. In addition, computer-based learning tools can emphasize lifelong learning (Zinatelli, Dube, & Jovanovic, 2002), a quality necessary to keep pace with the ever-changing client populations and cultures.

Previous computer experience and faculty promotion of software programs directly impacts student use (Thede, Taft, & Coeling, 1994). Previous computer experience may include degree of comfort and familiarity with computer use, satisfaction with software programs, correlation of CAI material with course content and immediate goals, self-efficacy about computer skills, easy access to CAI, satisfaction, and support services associated with CAI use. For example, the quality of the software program can influence student learning, interest, and motivation. A high-quality program is one that is interactive, stimulating, uses multimedia format, permits user control, and enables immediate and descriptive feedback in questioning (Khoiny, 1995). If software programs are to be perceived as user friendly, programs must be promoted consistently by faculty throughout the curriculum, beginning students must be introduced to CAI early in the curriculum, and software programs must complement and enhance learning via other educational media (e.g., film, video, reading, lecture). Using a standardized, reliable, and valid evaluation tool for appraising instructional software can enhance the probability that programs will meet overall curricular objectives (Boyce & Winne, 2000). Adding several items that evaluate the capacity to enhance learning related to cultural competence development and accurate exposure to multicultural clients, families, communities, nurses, and health care professionals will provide comparative information. Such data will help with purchasing decisions, design of strategies to integrate programs systematically throughout the course (and curriculum), and development of supplementary materials as needed to further address cultural similarities and differences. Examples of strategy design innovations are presented in Box 5.3.

Box 5.3   Innovations in cultural competence education:
Computer-assisted instruction

Sample Programmed Instruction Guide
  1. Click on the icon "Medical–Surgical Nursing."

2. Click on the case study "Care of the Client with _____."
3. Click on the CAI program option "Video with tutorial" and view segment 1.
4. What assumptions did you make about the client's cultural background in video segment 1? Why?
5. What assumptions did you make about the nurse's cultural background in video segment 1? Why?
6. What are the dangers of making assumptions based on physical characteristics, age, and/or gender?
7. Proceed to the video segment and tutorial CAI in segments 2–7.
8. What verbal and nonverbal communication techniques do the clients use?
9. What verbal and nonverbal communication techniques do the nurses use?
10. Are the communication patterns used effective? Why or why not?
11. What information concerning the client's cultural values, beliefs, and practices were presented?
12. How did the nurse incorporate the client's cultural values, beliefs, and practices into the plan of care?
13. To achieve culturally congruent care, what (else) should the nurse have done? Why?
14. Reflect on the traditional elderly Chinese client presented in last week's class video. How would the nurse–client interaction and plan of care be the same (or different) to achieve culturally congruent care? Explain.
15. Reflect on the case study about the Mexican American migrant worker presented in this week's assigned reading (chapter 12). How would the nurse–client interaction and plan of care be the same to achieve culturally congruent care? Explain.
16. Proceed to video segment and tutorial CAI numbers 8–15.
17. To achieve culturally congruent care, how would the nurse's discharge teaching and home care plan be the same (or different), if the client held the dominant (traditional) values, beliefs, and practices consistent with the _____ culture. (Examples: Egyptian, Filipino Italian, Nigerian, Lakota, Jamaican). Explain.
18. To achieve culturally congruent care, how would the nurse's discharge teaching and home care plan be the same (or different) if the client in the previously listed ethnic groups were also _____. (Examples: female, Muslim, Jehovah's Witness, Catholic, Jewish, Mormon, indigent, wealthy, illiterate, deaf, unemployed, unmarried). Explain.
19. Proceed to complete the review questions, and check your answers and rationale.
20. Reflect on your experience completing this CAI and programmed instruction guide questions. What did you like best? Discuss.

Unfortunately, the growing numbers of minority students and new immigrants in higher education have limited resources. Furthermore, limited access to computer technology will be characteristic of many minority and lower-income students (Burr, Burr, & Novak, 1999). The "nontraditional" student is older with multiple role responsibilities competing with academic demands; their organized study time and ability to use educational resources is often limited. Frequently, students are inefficacious in their ability to use computers and other educational resources. Consequently, integrating computer technology throughout the nursing curriculum must be accompanied by strategies to enhance nursing students' computer technology access, skills, use, and values (Jeffreys, 2004).

Unless CAI is valued and expected (required) throughout the curriculum, many students opt out of the "optional" CAI programs. Unfortunately, this will create a greater gap between those students who are computer literate or computer comfortable, and the potential values of CAI will never be realized. Faculty-run workshops at the beginning of each nursing course, designed to introduce small groups of students to CAI use, functions, and benefits should be supplemented by opportunities for short workshops throughout the semester and by advanced student peers and mentors. Adult learners respond best and are most motivated by perceived direct applicability to learning needs and long-term career goals. Highlighting the benefits within this context and introducing students to CAI programs most relevant to the current course will reap the greatest results. Results can be maximized by providing a warm, relaxed environment or place for students to use CAI, such as a nursing student resource center in which peer mentors (advanced students) serve as role models, resources, and guides to less advanced students (Jeffreys, 2004).

Web Page

The course web page has a unique opportunity to expand students' horizons in cultural competence development beyond geographic limitations. Because there are no geographic boundaries in cyberspace, students have the opportunity to venture out into worlds previously foreign, unknown, and undiscovered. Although the advantages are many, there are also disadvantages. One of the biggest disadvantages is that inaccurate information can be transmitted widely. Discriminating between reputable and reliable sites and questionable sites is often confusing to the novice (Andrews, Burr, & Janetos, 2004). Assisting students to access scholarly and reliable sites related to culture, health care, and nursing is an essential responsibility of educators. One way to do this is to create a course or program web page with direct links to reputable Internet sites and peer-reviewed professional literature (Xiao, 2005). Full-text journal articles increase access to reputable information. Web page features particularly important to the development of cultural competence are presented in Box 5.4.

Box 5.4   Innovations in cultural competence education:
Course web page

- Course
  announcements:

  Cultural events, holidays, meetings,
  conferences, food festival, newly published
  articles, discussion board invitation, brown
  bag roundtable discussion lunch meeting,
  check other part of web page

- Graphics, Photos,
  Slides

  Culturally diverse clients, students, nurses,
  and other health care providers in various
  settings. Graphics describing picture, event,
  date, individuals

- Virtual Tour

  Campus, nursing student resource center,
  nursing skills lab, depicting culturally
  diverse students, faculty, and staff

- Video Clip

  Previous examples

- Calendar

  Cultural holidays and events

- How to Use Web
  Page

  General information about blackboard
  features, support services for students who
  need assistance online, workshops, in-person
  support at nursing student resource center or
  college library/computer lab center, finding
  web page resources related to cultural
  competence

- Web Site Links:

  Local cultural agencies and resources, Ethnic
  Nursing Organizations, Transcultural
  Nursing Society (TCNS), local TCNS
  Chapter, Healthy People 2010, Office of
  Minority Health, U.S. Census, patient
  education

- Full-Text Articles

  Organized by cultural group (CINAHL,
  ERIC, Psychlit)

- Discussion Board

  Weekly discussion (asynchronous or
  synchronous) about a cultural clinical case
  study, assigned reading, video,
  computer-assisted instructional program, or
  other course component or outside assigned
  activity

- Reading
  Assignments

  Questions posted to prompt reflection and
  guide reading concerning to address cultural
  competency development

- Course
  Documents
Highlight cultural components in yellow for the following documents: course outline, program outcomes, characteristics of the graduate, Code of Ethics from ANA, ICN, NSNA.
Transcultural Nursing Code of Ethics, National Standards for Culturally and Linguistically Appropriate Services in Health Care

- E-Mail
Individual, select, and all user communication to send personalized messages in addition to course announcements

---

Students, especially nontraditional students, will need ongoing guidance about computer technology, literature and web searches, and the computer-assistance services available via the nursing department and the college (Mertig, 2003). By enhancing the ease with which students can access known reputable information, students can become more confident (efficacious) about developing their transcultural nursing skills. For example, a student who retrieves known reputable information about a particular cultural group and clinical topic will be better prepared to conduct a culturally congruent health history in the clinical setting and most likely will be realistically efficacious. Optimally, a workshop designed and conducted by the course instructor, librarian, or nursing support personnel will maximize student use by increasing knowledge, computer skills, and appreciation of computer technology (Xiao, 2005). Often, students are inefficacious about computer skills, library searches, or resources available. Strategies that expand on instructor workshops, especially ones that incorporate peer mentors and role modeling, will enhance student use, persistence, satisfaction, and self-efficacy concerning computer use and research skills (Jeffreys, 2004).

Nursing Skills Laboratory

Traditionally, the main purpose of the nursing skills laboratory (NSL) was to permit the teaching and practicing of clinical skills via a non-threatening, controlled environment and simulation. *Simulation* has been defined as a situation or event made to resemble clinical practice (Rauen, 2001). Simulation permits the student to practice clinical skills prior to implementation on a real patient. Whether the NSL contains the new high-technology human patient simulators, simulated patient actors, or rubber mannequins, it is simulation as a teaching method that has much potential in enhancing learning. Simulation can increase knowledge, critical thinking, and confidence; it has been used successfully in nursing education for clinical skills (Medley & Horne, 2005; Morton & Rauen, 2004; Nehring & Lashley, 2004; Ulrich & Glendon, 1999).

Nurse educators have a wonderful opportunity to further develop students' cultural competence by creating simulated patient case scenarios that incorporate cultural dimensions. Simulated patient case scenarios build self-efficacy, critical thinking, and clinical decision making (Dearman, 2003). First, the NSL environment can be modeled (or remodeled) to outwardly embrace and emphasize cultural diversity. Although the purchase of culturally diverse mannequins may be one option, the market options for mannequins are limited to a few differences in physical characteristics, neglecting the more important variations in CVB. There are more detailed and inexpensive strategies to make the NSL more "culturally friendly" and inclusive. For example, each rubber mannequin can be given a name and background information representing different ethnic, racial, gender, socioeconomic, age, and religious groups. Corresponding patient charts, bed tags, patient identification tags, ethnic clothing, religious articles, non-English reading materials, ethnic menus, and other items can be placed on or near the mannequins. Clinical case scenarios, incorporating various cultural data along with the clinical topics relevant to previous class sessions and the current week's class, can be developed into a large-group discussion, small-group activity, role play, case exemplar, care plan, and/or other learner-centered activity.

As with any teaching strategy, it will be beneficial to explain the purpose, objectives, activities, and time frame before the onset. Supplementing verbal information with a brief outline or handout can be used as a reference for students periodically throughout the activity to keep students on target. A debriefing session will help summarize and clarify key points, giving the nurse educator another opportunity to emphasize cultural competence development as an expected component to any clinical skill. To further enhance affective learning and self-discovery (as well as provide feedback to the nurse educator), students can be asked to reflect on the case scenario, group discussion, or other activity. Written student comments and feedback will provide new insight into the teaching strategy's perceived benefits, limitations, and learning associated with furthering cultural competence development; student feedback will be valuable in modifying or continuing with strategy components.

Other strategies for making the NSL "culturally friendly" and inclusive extend toward making culturally diverse students feel welcome. NSL posters, bulletin boards, and journal article postings that celebrate cultural diversity and emphasize the nursing professional's role in cultural-specific nursing care is one strategy. Creating situational questions that address cultural issues as new clinical skills are introduced, or previously learned skills are refreshed to supplement and enhance learning.

Awareness that covert or subtle racism can consciously or unconsciously create feelings of isolation, stress, and cultural pain must also acknowledge that these unwanted feelings can adversely influence learning. One example of subtle racism in nursing and health care is the prevalence of physical examination "norms" that are based on the assessment of a "white" individual (Barbee & Gibson, 2001). Discussing and demonstrating physical assessment skills to accurately assess patients with dark skin pigmentation for stage I decubiti, cyanosis, jaundice, petechiae, Kaposi's sarcoma, melanoma, and other assessments should be integrated as an expected component within the appropriate clinical topics; these assessment skills should not be presented as an afterthought.

Prior to the implementation of skills with patients in clinical settings, students may be observed or tested to assure a minimum level of proficiency. Although the purpose of the NSL is to enhance learning and develop confidence via a nonthreatening environment, the testing and retesting of nursing skills can greatly increase stress, thereby decreasing learning and satisfaction (Delgado & Mack, 2002). This is particularly true if students' CVB perceive learning performance to be a direct reflection on the teacher, demanding proficiency and excellence after initial instructor demonstration. Nurse educators must learn to adapt teaching styles to accommodate students' diverse CVB concerning learning and the teacher–student role if culturally congruent teaching is to be achieved. Culturally congruent teaching–learning strategies must be integrated within all components of nursing education. Table 5.2 presents several examples contrasting culturally congruent and culturally incongruent teacher–student interactions. Creating a caring, nurturing community through "care groups" for enhancing cognitive, psychomotor, and affective learning in the NSL is one successfully implemented strategy (Pullen, Murray, & McGee, 2001, 2003).

Clinical Settings

Although great differences in types of clinical settings, learning experiences, and instructor involvement exists, there are certain criteria that should be considered. One consideration is the clinical setting's cultural diversity of clients, nurses, and other agency personnel in relation to the surrounding community and to the nursing student population. A second consideration involves students' perceptions concerning diversity. Routine collection and analysis of data from a "student evaluation of clinical

Table 5.2   Faculty Helpfulness in the Nursing Skills Laboratory, Clinical Setting, and Classroom: Examples of Culturally Incongruent and Culturally Congruent Approaches

Situation	Culturally Incongruent	Culturally Congruent
Nursing Skills Laboratory		
After a detailed skills laboratory class on injections, it is now Lee's turn to administer an intramuscular injection into the skills laboratory mannequin for the first time. Lee's CVB view the teacher as an authority figure. Less than perfect performance would poorly reflect on the teacher and cause embarrassment for the teacher in front of the other students. Lee is fearful that she will not demonstrate the skill perfectly and feels that she must "save face"; yet, Lee does not want to refuse the professor's request to "inject." Anxiously, she asks if she can first practice with her peers.	Professor wants to help all students equally and aims to "treat all students alike." Professor insists that Lee administer the injection. *Result:* Lee feels increasingly anxious and pressured that she must perform the injection perfectly. In addition, she feels cultural pain because she believes that she initiated conflict with an authority figure. Lee attempts the injection, but when she forgets to aspirate, she becomes even more anxious and experiences cultural pain because she has now "embarrassed her teacher." Lee feels much dissatisfaction and stress; she questions her ability to complete the nursing program.	Professor recognizes that Lee's anxiety may not be related to lack of academic readiness but rather to underlying CVB. Professor reassures Lee that she does not expect perfection on the first attempt; however, she still notes nonverbal cues of anxiety (facial tension, shaking hands, flushed appearance). Professor pairs Lee with a strong student who has already performed the injection and allows privacy for several practice injections. *Result:* Lee does not feel pressured to "save face" and can relax enough with her peer to perfect her skill prior to observation by the instructor. After demonstrating the injection to the professor accurately, Lee experiences satisfaction.
Clinical		
During clinical postconference, one student (Jane) assertively questions the clinical instructor's statement about a medication. Jane's CVB openly encourage assertiveness and	Professor's CVB consider the preservation of group harmony and "saving face" as a priority. She sees the discomfort of two other students in the group and aims to help the group avoid	Professor recognizes differences between individual orientation versus group orientation. Although her own CVB are group orientation, Professor realizes that Jane's behavior is *(continued)*

Table 5.2 (*Continued*)

Situation	Culturally Incongruent	Culturally Congruent
equally view teachers and learners as coparticipants in the teaching–learning process. Several students with different CVB are obviously uncomfortable by the perceived confrontation.	conflict. Professor's response is to evade answering Jane's question and dismiss the postconference early. *Result:* Jane is still confused and feels stressed about the medication. She is dissatisfied with the professor's actions.	appropriate. Professor answers Jane's question and uses this opportunity to discuss various differences in communication patterns, values, and beliefs among different cultures. *Result:* Jane and the other students receive clarification about the statement and receive new information about culture and values clarification, enhancing academic outcomes and promoting positive psychological outcomes.
Classroom		
Lou performed excellently on an exam, achieving the highest grade. Lou has group orientation rather than individual orientation; therefore, he is uncomfortable with individual praise.	Professor intends to be helpful, acknowledge strong performance, and motivate other students. Professor verbally praises Lou's performance in the classroom, announcing his name and exceptional performance. *Result:* Lou is embarrassed and feels ashamed over being singled out in the class.	Professor intends to be helpful and acknowledges strong performance and motivates other students; yet, she is aware of CVB that affect a culturally congruent approach. Professor verbally acknowledges the outstanding performance demonstrated by several students without mentioning their names. *Result:* Lou feels satisfied and comfortable with the knowledge that his performance and that of others in the group has been appreciated.

Adapted from Jeffreys, M. R. (2004). *Nursing student retention: Understanding the process and making a difference.* New York, Springer. Used by permission, Springer Publishing Company, Inc., New York 10036.

experience" questionnaire can provide valuable insight, especially if items solicit information concerning client characteristics and the students' perception about the clinical setting's cultural diversity (Jeffreys, Massoni, O'Donnell, & Smodlaka, 1997).

Interaction with cultural diverse patients, families, communities, and health care providers in the clinical setting offers a wealth of learning opportunities for students. Providing opportunities for students to interact with cultural diverse clients and personnel must be appropriately partnered with cultural competence development as an integral course and curricular component. Students must have the general transcultural nursing skills, knowledge, and values to successfully achieve positive learning outcomes for cultural competence development. As mentioned previously, TSE (confidence) perceptions will directly influence student's commitment, motivation, and persistence with transcultural skills. Because interactions may result in "cultural mistakes," inefficacious students may avoid cultural considerations when planning and implementing care. Overly confident students may never exercise the task of "preparing" to engage in culturally congruent patient interactions, assessments, planning, or interventions. Without appropriate guidance and feedback, students' TSE perceptions may adversely affect student learning, performance, and outcomes, as well as cause negative effects on patient care and patient outcomes (see Figure 2.2).

Initial and ongoing student assessment must include transcultural knowledge, skills, values, and confidence. Nurse educators can develop individual and group diagnostic-prescriptive educational interventions based on assessment findings. Anecdotal notes should include regular entries describing student strengths, weaknesses, and client description (Oermann & Gaberson, 1998; Schoolcraft & Novotny, 2000). Often, clinical instructors keep anecdotal notes detailing clinical skills or tasks performed by students' and patients' medical diagnoses. This information is then used to rotate students through various clinical skills, tasks, and medical diagnoses. A proactive action for enhancing cultural competence development expands anecdotal notes to include details about patient's cultural dimensions and the transcultural skills learned and/or performed by the student.

Clinical instructors have unlimited opportunities to effectively weave cultural competence development activities throughout the clinical learning experience. Although some learning experiences may be preplanned, clinical instructors must be prepared to be flexible and to adapt learning objectives to the ever-changing situation. Because the clinical setting is not a "controlled" environment, clinical instructors must always be ready to expect the unexpected. Unexpected situations will present new learning opportunities for student's professional growth; some of these unexpected situations may be rich opportunities for expanding cultural competence. Despite the cultural diversity within a clinical setting, the instructor is pivotal to guide students to new levels of cultural competence development. The clinical instructor can supplement actual clinical experiences with case studies representing different cultural groups, values, beliefs, behaviors, and/or practices. A guided postclinical conference whereby students work together or in small groups to critically appraise information and propose a culturally congruent plan of care is another option.

Preplanned learning objectives that incorporate cultural competence development may or may not be shared with students at the onset of the clinical experience. For example, if self-discovery or group learning through discovery is an intended outcome, telling students about the desired outcomes would be inappropriate. Guided discussion and shared information during a clinical postconference can help students discover the diverse patient groups represented that day and how similar or different CVB affected the implementation of culturally congruent nursing care, clinical skills, and actual/potential patient outcomes (see Education-in-Action Vignette Box 5.5). Postconference summary of student's cognitive, practical, and affective learning outcomes will be beneficial to future learning activities designed to incorporate this prerequisite learning. Besides comparison of the same clinical skill, other possibilities are cultural similarities and differences between patients with the same signs, symptoms, medical diagnoses, nursing diagnoses, diagnostic procedures, treatments, or prognoses. Positive, realistic instructor feedback and vicarious learning (by observing others) will help improve TSE perceptions.

In clinical settings where the clinical instructor is not present (e.g., home visits or internship), preset learning objectives that include cultural competence must be clearly delineated. Instructor comments on weekly journal entries, peer comments on course web page discussion boards, and/or postclinical conferences and seminars will further assist students connect experiences in their cultural competence development.

Positive learning experiences have been reported from immersion experiences or community placements (Cummings, 1998; Gomez & White, 2002; Haloburdo & Thompson, 1998; Kollar & Ailinger, 2002; Leininger & McFarland, 2002; Moch, Long, Jones, Shadlick, & Solheim, 1999; Pickerell, 2001; Ryan, Twibell, Brigham, & Bennett, 2000; St. Clair & McKenry, 1999; Stevens, 1998; Tabi & Mukherjee, 2003). Despite the reported benefits, it is crucial that immersion experiences in cultural communities or international clinical experiences are sufficiently linked with prerequisite and onsite comprehensive learning about the host culture. In addition, experiences should contain sufficient patient–nurse interaction and should be followed with reflective components to enhance long-term positive learning impact on students (Kollar & Ailinger, 2002; Leininger

& McFarland, 2002; St. Clair & McKenry, 1999). Adequate preparation and support during the immersion experience must incorporate effective coping strategies (Ryan et al., 2000).

Students can also benefit by the awareness that faculty are also learning and developing cultural competency skills within ethnic communities (Leininger & McFarland, 2002; Moch et al., 1999). By reaching out to surrounding communities, community-based curricula have the potential to provide students with a wealth of valuable experiences if accompanied by other substantial curricular components that embrace a wide diversity of cultures. "Tacking on" culture courses or course components or the "adopt a community" approach alone is insufficient for preparing nurses and nursing students to provide culturally congruent care (Baldwin, 1999).

Written assignments. Written assignments may be differentiated between low-stakes and high-stakes assignments. Each type has a potentially valuable role in cultural competence development, if used effectively. Low-stakes writing minimizes the pressure of "grading" associated with high-stakes writing (Elbow, 1997) and optimizes affective learning outcomes. Unfortunately, because low-stakes writing assignments have the potential to be unvalued or undervalued by both students and faculty, low-stakes writing assignments are often underused. Affective learning is an important component in cultural competence development; therefore, the design of carefully planned low-stakes writing assignments targeting cultural issues should be an integral component in various dimensions of the course (clinical, classroom, NSL, immersion components). Known teaching–learning strategies that strongly enhance affective learning must be incorporated within written assignments. Reflection is one strategy that enhances affective learning (Schön, 1987). Engaging the student via in-class or out-of-class written assignments can easily include an individual reflective component. For example, students can be asked to write a "low-stakes" written reflection about

- In-class group discussion about culturally competent ethical decision making for the assigned case study
- Feelings experienced after viewing a film on racism
- Changes in views on transcultural nursing since the beginning of the semester
- Feelings experienced before, during, and after interviewing a culturally different person about his or her cultural values, beliefs, and practices
- Changes in perceived confidence for providing culturally congruent care for culturally different patients

- New feelings of appreciation for cultural diversity within the nursing profession
- Most valuable learning from the process of completing a review of literature paper on a specific cultural group
- Feelings experienced after reading a journal article on health disparities and health care disparities among diverse populations

The benefits of transferring reflective thoughts into written format have the potential to further develop student's affective learning. The exercise of writing encourages students to reflect, organize, and synthesize thoughts before writing, thus assisting students in gaining new insights and self-discovery. Students can reread and then reflect on written ideas, thus leading to higher levels of thoughtful synthesized inquiry, reflection, insight, and learning. The nurse educator who skillfully reviews written low-stakes writing assignments has the unique benefit of gaining insight into another dimension of student's thought process, learning, beliefs, values, strengths, weaknesses, and confidence. Nurse educator's positive written feedback and nonthreatening written questions serve to further guide or mentor students' affective learning and cultural competence development. For example, mentored clinical journals have been identified to enhance the process of reflection and critical thinking (Bilinski, 2002); such an approach can be adapted to focus students on cultural-specific care and issues. Preparing a series of questions and objectives for written journal reflections can assist students in their self-discovery experienced during an immersion experience (Gomez & White, 2002; St. Clair & McKenry, 1999).

High-stakes written assignments or papers have the potential to achieve positive learning outcomes if strategically linked with other course components. Unfortunately, many students (and some educators) view written papers such as term papers as a final end product. The real value of a written assignment is the process of completing the assignment rather than the mere product (paper). Such a philosophy corresponds with the writing-to-learn (WTL) strategy in which various in-class and out-of-class writing activities aim to further develop thinking and learning over an extended period of time (Schmidt, 2004a, 2004b). For example, written term papers that can and are completed in 1 to 2 days, rather than over an extended period, do not achieve desirable outcomes. Exhaustion, dislike, and short-term memory predominate, hindering the long-term goal of building a repertoire of skills, values, and knowledge needed for developing cultural competence and confidence.

If a written assignment is to have any real effect on the ongoing development of cultural competence, then the emphasis of the assignment should be on the process of completing the assignment. Elements that favor the achievement of long-term learning outcomes include

- Stagger over a period of time with periodic in-class discussion over the process of the paper
- Link with other course components and course topics
- Demonstrate evidence of long-term benefits to student's future professional role
- Distribute a written guide to the "process" of completing the assignment
- Collect drafts or portions of the paper throughout the semester and provide constructive feedback
- Integrate several different learning activities
- Include a reflective component that targets affective learning
- Define evaluative criteria with appropriately weighted grading distribution components
- Publicize easily accessible resources for completing the assignment

Within the context of papers aimed at cultural issues and developing cultural competence, long-term effects plus the potential for expanding knowledge, skills, and values through synthesis is desirable. This involves commitment, time, and coordinated planning among faculty in an effort to link various approaches. One example, an innovative philosophy for creative learning activities called "cultural discovery," included a written paper assignment in conjunction with several other components. Background reading assignments, classroom activity components (lecture and discussion), clinical postconference discussions, a collaborative library introductory program, a videotape program, an interview of a culturally different elderly person, a cultural assessment, Leininger's Acculturation Health Care Assessment Enabler for Cultural Patterns in Traditional and Nontraditional Lifeways (Leininger, 1991c) a literature review, and a reflection were used. "Cultural discovery" assisted first-semester associate's degree students to systematically conduct a basic cultural assessment, identify similarities and differences among individuals within cultural groups, distinguish between varying dimensions of acculturation, discover the importance of culturally congruent nursing care, and recognize cultural competence development as an ongoing process (Jeffreys & O'Donnell, 1997). The "process" of the written assignment was multidimensional with various learner-centered activities connecting clinical and classroom topics and incorporating cognitive, psychomotor/practical (communication), and affective skills. The "product" of the written assignment (paper) provided concrete evidence of the connection between the components.

Weekly written care plans that incorporate cultural assessment data into the plan of care is another strategy to develop cultural competence. A written weekly journal and then a summary journal entry focusing on cultural issues and culturally congruent care can provide a measure of type of cognitive, practical, and affective learning within the context of cultural competence development. Written reports following observational experiences in various settings with clients of different ethnic, racial, cultural, and socioeconomic groups is another approach. Every written assignment has the potential to have a cultural component integrated substantially within it. One important question is "Does it?" A second question is "How is the cultural component piece perceived by students?" Inclusion of a reflective component, an anonymous survey with open-ended questions and/or comment section, and/or focus groups will provide nurse educators with valuable information about student perceptions and learning that can guide strategy modifications.

Because adult learners are most motivated to engage in activities that they perceive are most relevant, it is important to truly capture the students' interest in the written paper. For example, many students enrolled in a master's program with an adult health clinical nurse specialist (CNS) focus do not enter the master's program with the primary goal of developing cultural competency. Typically, CNS students are interested in developing clinical competencies in a clinical specialty and obtaining certification in a clinical specialty; therefore, nurse educators are challenged to invigorate zeal and instill interest among these adult learners. A foundational required course in transcultural nursing offers the best approach because students will similarly be introduced to the knowledge, skills, and values for developing cultural competence (Jeffreys, 2002; Leininger, 1995b). To capture student's interest and to develop cultural competencies at the CNS level, students enrolled in a required transcultural core course in the CNS curriculum were asked to write two papers that would help develop the selected area of the adult health CNS role (Jeffreys, 2002). The following strategies assisted students with the process of writing and with conducting a review of literature on cultural and clinical topics:

- The "Guide to Writing" handbook included strategies for selecting topics, narrowing topics, writing an introduction, method of literature search, synthesizing ideas, and so on
- Course web page contained bibliography and links to relevant cultural and clinical resources

- Weekly (brief) end-of-class group discussion concerning process of assignment and ongoing reflection
- Individual or small-group meetings with instructor as needed
- Submission of designated paper components over the semester
- Incorporation of instructor comments into revision

Sharing information during the process of writing assisted students with developing knowledge, skills, and values necessary for cultural competent advanced practice nursing, writing, and research. During the graduate seminars, students discussed the "lived experience" about the process involved with the paper. Peers as role models presented both the achievements and struggles; vicarious learning and role modeling can effectively increase self-efficacy, motivation, learning, and persistence (Bandura, 1986). Disseminating information to others after "product" or paper is completed helps synthesize information and broadens the learning beyond one's own research and paper to gain insight into other perspectives, recognizing similarities and differences within and between cultural groups. Dissemination may be done via newsletter, journal, web site, video, oral presentation, poster presentation, and/or PowerPoint presentation.

Presentations

The presentations discussed in this chapter include oral, poster, and PowerPoint presentation. Individually or in combination with each other, these types of presentation have great power in disseminating information, views, skills, feelings, attitudes, and resources about cultural competence that can positively influence cultural competence and confidence. Nurse educators need to be astute in guiding students so stereotypes and misperceptions are not perpetuated intentionally or inadvertently. For example, if an undergraduate "introduction to research" small-group class assignment includes reading a research article, preparing a poster, and presenting orally to the class, students should be reminded to mention study limitations, especially sampling and generalizability. Although the main focus of the research class is understanding the steps of the research process, critically appraising research for utilization in clinical practice and identifying areas for further research, nurse educators have many creative opportunities for introducing cultural issues related to research. One approach may be that several presentations include any one or more of the following combinations:

- Different methodology with the same cultural group
- Same methodology with different cultural groups

- Same research topic with different cultural groups
- Same methodology with the same cultural group but different socioeconomic status, gender, or age
- Different conceptual frameworks and same cultural group
- Same conceptual framework and different cultural groups

Allocating brief question/answer and comment sessions after each presentation permits students to clarify information and feelings, as well as to discover similarities and differences within and between groups. A summary dialog and discussion can further compare and contrast information about cultures.

To enhance cultural learning while also promoting positive feelings about the overall "presentation" experience, several additional strategies may be employed. The sharing of cultural foods, beverages, and music of presented cultural groups promotes sensory stimulation and learning through sight, taste, touch, smell, and sound. Compilation of presenters' abstracts into a professional looking "Book of Abstracts" organized alphabetically by cultural group, topic, or presenter provides a mechanism for ongoing networks, shared information, long-term learning, and validation. Opportunities for students to display posters or present information at a nursing student club meeting, professional meeting, recruitment event, local ethnic nursing meeting, Transcultural Nursing Society local chapter meeting, or Sigma Theta Tau chapter meeting is beneficial for the audience and for the presenters. Professional events that encourage students' active participation offer students validation for their achievements so far in their professional development and their educational process. Validation is important and helps increase self-efficacy. Validation is especially important for nontraditional students (older, commuter, and/or minority) and has been positively linked with persistence behaviors (Rendon, 1994; Rendon, Jalomo, & Nora, 2000). Students who are recognized and thanked by members of the professional community for their presentation, as well as for their time, receive positive feedback for their professional nursing actions to enhance cultural competence development in self and in others.

Exams

Unfortunately, many students associate the importance of learning and information based on what will be on an upcoming exam. Multiple-choice test questions, short answer exam questions, and/or essay questions concerning culturally congruent care have the potential to further demonstrate the importance of cultural competence and to provide valuable feedback about learning (and teaching). A quantitative award (test item points or test grade) that directly impacts the course grade validates cultural competence as significant enough to award a quantitative measure that will affect the immediate course grade and progression in the nursing curriculum. In contrast, testing in which cultural diversity and cultural competence is invisible may inadvertently reinforce students' misperception that cultural competence is nonessential, cosmetic, optional, irrelevant, or a time waster. Furthermore, absence of testing results in the lack of empirical data necessary to identify learner strengths and weaknesses, guide teaching–learning interventions, and direct course and curricular revision.

Views on testing, type of testing, and comfort and familiarity with different test formats and procedures varies among culturally diverse and academically diverse students. Assessing students' familiarity with test formats, concerns, anxiety, confidence, strengths, weaknesses, and past test experiences is a necessary first step when designing culturally congruent test items and exams. A general overview of learner characteristics within the student cohort group provides valuable information (see Box 5.1 and Table 1.2). Although the topic of testing is quite complicated, several key considerations are mentioned in this chapter. First, students with primary and/or secondary education in foreign countries may be unfamiliar with multiple-choice questions, especially those that require decision making and critical thinking. Some foreign-educated individuals are more familiar with essay questions or questions requiring rote memorization. Second, students educated within at-risk school districts within the United States are at risk for poor test-taking skills and low confidence for taking exams. Third, older students or students with substantial gaps in their educational experience may benefit from "refresher" techniques for taking tests. Fourth, multiple-choice exams may require a different approach to thinking and communicating than typically used within the students' cultural group. Finally, exams should be free of overt and covert cultural biases. For example, among traditional Native American students, Crow (1993) recommended incorporating both individual and family into the keyed multiple-choice response rather than demanding that a choice be made between family and individual.

It is challenging to create exams that are fair, valid, and culturally congruent with respect to cultural knowledge, skills, and values tested, as well as to the culturally diverse learner. Offering test preparation workshops periodically throughout the semester and incorporating learner characteristics and ongoing assessments into the workshops can make a positive difference by enhancing learning, test success, and confidence. Recognizing that students' responses to types of instructor feedback may vary based on CVB, nurse educators are challenged to develop culturally congruent approaches for advice, feedback, helpfulness, and recognition (see Table 5.2).

Workshops can identify additional strengths, weaknesses, and gaps, thereby providing valuable information to guide subsequent workshops and teaching strategies within this student cohort and future student groups. As part of the formative evaluation, administration of a workshop evaluation survey after each workshop will provide feedback concerning students' perceptions. A summative evaluation may include administration of a survey to evaluate students' perceptions about test preparation workshops and test-taking skills at the end of the semester, year, and/or program.

Supplementary Resources

Within the academic setting, supplementary resources have the potential to support or restrict cultural competence development. Examples of supplementary resources include the library, enrichment programs (EPs), nursing student resource center (NSRC), nursing student club (NSC), bulletin boards, local Sigma Theta Tau International (STTI) Honor Society in Nursing Chapter, local chapters of specialty and ethnic nursing associations, and invited guest speakers. Resources that embrace cultural diversity by being culturally friendly and inclusive of culturally diverse and academically diverse nursing students create caring environments that foster student feelings of social integration, satisfaction, and cultural congruence with the nursing profession and educational institution. For example, the aforementioned supplementary resources outwardly display a celebration of diversity if respective brochures, posters, mentors, employees, workshops, invited guest speakers, events, meetings, and student participants appropriately represent various cultural groups.

Appraising existing supplementary resources beyond their superficial appearance may uncover untapped areas necessitating further action, expansion, inclusiveness, and innovation. Similarly, the discovery that supplementary resources do not exist suggests the need for immediate action and innovation. Several ideas follow:

- Develop collaborative partnerships with librarians.
- Obtain new library resources for cultural competence development.
- Foster cross-cultural student interaction via EP study groups led by peer mentor-tutors.
- Revise NSRC brochures to feature students of different age, gender, and cultural groups.

- Advertise upcoming cultural events, holidays, and workshops on bulletin boards.
- Host an international food festival organized by the NSC.
- Co-sponsor a cultural workshop with STTI chapter and involve students as volunteers.
- Sponsor student(s) for participation in cultural nursing conference.
- Establish networks with local ethnic nursing associations.
- Form a local chapter of the transcultural nursing society.
- Raffle a student membership in the Transcultural Nursing Society and local chapter.
- Invite guest speakers from different cultural backgrounds to speak about cultural topics.

Nurse educators are challenged to expand the web of student inclusion beyond the traditionally required educational curriculum and setting through professional events and memberships. The web of inclusion refers to an interwoven professional network that embraces culturally diverse students and strives to promote professional integration and cultural competence development through participation in professional events and memberships (Jeffreys, 2004). Participation in professional events and memberships is viewed as an essential activity for professional growth and career mobility by providing unique opportunities for professional socialization, networking, skill enhancement, knowledge expansion, and professional attitude development (Betts & Cherry, 2002; Joel & Kelly, 2002). Strategies that enhance student opportunities to actively use supplementary resources and participate in cultural competence development outside of nursing courses will ultimately benefit both students and the nursing profession.

KEY POINT SUMMARY

- The academic setting has the potential to make enormous strides in cultural competence development, especially through entry-level education.
- Cultural competence development can only occur with well-qualified, committed nursing faculty and through the use of culturally congruent teaching–learning strategies that address students' diverse cultural values and beliefs (CVB).
- Each individual faculty member is empowered to make a positive difference; however, the greatest impact will be achieved through a coordinated, holistic group effort that thoughtfully weaves

together nursing course components, nursing curriculum, and supplementary resources.

- Promoting cultural competency in academia requires considerable, sincere effort that begins with faculty self-assessment.
- Resilient TSE (confidence) is the integral component necessary in the process of cultural competence development (of self and in others).
- Resilient TSE perceptions embrace lifelong learning in the quest to become "more" culturally competent and in the quest to assist others (learners) to become more culturally competent.
- At the undergraduate and graduate setting, it becomes increasingly urgent to closely examine how visible (or invisible) cultural competency development is actively present.
- Examination at the curricular, program, school, and course level requires courage, commitment, time, energy, and a systematic plan.
- Inquiry, action, and innovation at the curriculum level involve the philosophy, conceptual framework, program objectives, program outcomes, courses, course components, horizontal threads, and vertical threads.
- Inquiry, action, and innovation at the course level involve the course outline, instructional media, learning activities, course components, and clinical settings.
- Inquiry, action, and innovation at the supplementary resource level involves the library, enrichment programs, nursing student clubs, nursing student resource center, bulletin boards, honor society chapter, local organizations, and guest speakers.
- Cultural competence development must be introduced early, integrated purposely, and intricately woven within the academic setting to create a durable fabric that provides long-lasting learning and desirable educational, professional, and patient outcomes.

Box 5.5   Educator-in-Action Vignette

As part of the preclinical conference, Professor Hart mentions that several students will administer digoxin orally to the patients. Through guided questioning, Professor Hart assists students in discussing and reviewing key information and nursing implications associated with digoxin administration.

Dawn says, "I know it is important to assess the apical pulse for 1 full minute. If the pulse is regular and at least 60 beats/minute, I will give the digoxin to my patient. The drug handbook mentioned to also check serum digoxin levels first."

All students agree that these are the most important assessments when administering digoxin.

Professor Hart has purposely selected several culturally diverse patients and reminds students to incorporate culture into the plan of care. She hopes that through self-discovery, students will realize significance of culture within all aspects of patient care. Professor Hart plans to assist students as needed throughout the patient care experience and during the clinical postconference.

After preclinical conference, Dawn quietly says to Steven, "I don't know why Professor Hart always stresses culture so much. Most parts of nursing care can just be done as described in the procedure book. Besides, how many ways can you give an oral medication?"

Student excerpts from clinical postconference are listed:

Steven: My patient was a 64-year-old female who was a religious Muslim from Pakistan. When I told her that it was important to listen to her heart before giving her the heart medication, she said she did not want to take her pill and became upset. When I asked her if she would prefer a female nursing student to listen to her heart, she was agreeable. After a few minutes, Janice assessed the apical rate and administered the medication with Professor Hart observing.

Janice: Yes, I also learned that it was important to use my right hand to place the digoxin in her mouth and offer her water using my right hand. She needed my help because she had bilateral arm casts.

Dawn: My patient was a 75-year-old recent immigrant from China who spoke some English. Her heart rate was 72. When I brought her the digoxin to take with a cold glass of water, she did not want to take the pill. The nurse explained that consistent with traditional Chinese beliefs, my patient preferred warm beverages. When I brought her some hot tea, she readily took her digoxin. I guess I was overly confident about how easy it would be to administer medications without realizing cultural beliefs and customs could really make a difference. Next time, I will try to prepare better.

Katie: I had a similar experience. My patient would only take her medication with grapefruit juice. She told me that in Puerto Rico grapefruit juice is quite popular to promote health. After checking that there were no interactions between grapefruit juice, digoxin, and her other medications, I provided her with some juice.

Juanita: My patient also had digoxin ordered. He did not want to take anything by mouth because it is a religious "fast" day. With my patient's permission, I contacted the hospital priest to speak with him. Afterward, my patient was so happy because he also got to receive Communion. The priest explained that it was okay to take medication orally.

Professor Hart encouraged questions and elaborated on the various customs and beliefs "discovered" by the students. She provided students with some additional examples using different cultural groups, reminding students to individually appraise each patient to avoid stereotypes. At the end of the discussion, Professor Hart asked students to reflect and write about their most important learning experiences. Review of the written reflections would guide her on future assignments, teaching–learning strategies, and students' cultural competence development. Written feedback, returned to students the following week, would provide encouragement and guidance to continue on their journey for culturally congruent patient care.

CHAPTER 6

Health Care Institutions

Health care institutions (HCIs) are in a unique position to both encourage and expect ongoing cultural competence development and culturally congruent patient care (see Figure 6.1). Expectations must be partnered with structured, high-quality educational opportunities and incentives for enhancing cultural competence development that are motivated by true commitment for cultural competence rather than by accrediting agency mandates. Because cultural competence is defined as a multidimensional learning process that integrates transcultural skills in all three dimensions (cognitive, practical, and affective) and involves transcultural self-efficacy (TSE) (confidence) as a major influencing factor, high-quality opportunities must be carefully planned and coordinated to integrate these components. The term *learning process* emphasizes that the cognitive, practical, and affective dimensions of TSE and transcultural skill development can change over time as a result of formalized education and other learning experiences.

Although informal interaction within the HCI can provide contact with other cultures that can have valuable and positive learning outcomes, especially if supplemented with appropriate formalized educational experiences, unguided interactions can unintentionally perpetrate stereotypes and misperceptions. One common misperception is that one member of a particular cultural group is the authority or example for all aspects of the group's values, beliefs, and practices; hence, stereotyping may ensue. Another common misperception is that being a member of a minority group automatically makes one the authority on cultural competence for minority group(s) and on the process of promoting cultural competency development in others. Contrary to this unfounded belief, scholars support that all individuals, regardless of cultural background, need formalized preparation in transcultural nursing—at least on the generalist level (Andrews, 1995; Leininger, 1995b; Leininger & McFarland, 2002).

116

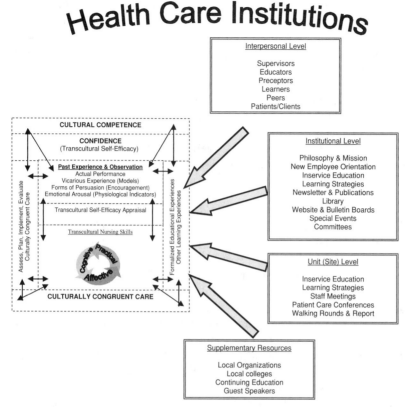

Figure 6.1   Health care institutions.

Preparation on the generalist level emphasizes broad transcultural nursing principles, concepts, theories, and research study findings to care for clients of many different cultures (Leininger, 1989).

Learners will be most motivated and interested in learning whether immediate benefits to career goals and daily professional responsibilities are clearly evident and whether learning goals are realistic (Brookfield, 1986; Knowles, 1984). With increased globalization and the changing demographics and characteristics within and between cultural groups, it is unrealistic to expect that nurses will become specialists in caring for (or working with) the many different cultural groups they may encounter. To become a specialist in one or more select cultural groups requires a series of specialized transcultural courses and concentrated fieldwork at the graduate level (Leininger, 1989; Leininger & McFarland, 2002). Although this type of formalized education occurs in an academic setting, the HCI has an important role in facilitating nurses' advanced degrees. The HCI may provide incentives (flexible scheduling, promotions, released time, tuition reimbursement, forgivable loans, certified transcultural nurse certification fee and expenses) for nurses to become advanced practice nurses as transcultural nurse specialists. Transcultural nurse specialists will be valuable resources within the HCI and the surrounding cultural community. It is realistic to expect that all nurses have the basic or generalist transcultural nursing skills needed to provide care for culturally diverse and different clients. It is also reasonable to expect nurses who have been prepared as generalists to participate in ongoing educational programs designed to expand their learning with direct application to specific, targeted priority cultural groups in the surrounding communities.

Because few nurses have had formal preparation in transcultural nursing at entry into practice and because not all nurses will pursue higher education, the HCI assumes a great responsibility for assuring the public that nurses are prepared to provide culturally congruent care and that the care is appropriately rendered. Unfortunately, heightened patient acuity levels, the nursing shortage, poor nurse retention, inadequate staffing, rapidly changing culturally diverse patient populations, managed care, and limited resources create numerous, ongoing challenges for HCIs. First, patient care activities often must compete with educational programs. Second, providing ongoing education programs for nurses passing through a revolving door system of changing positions, units, agencies, and shifts presents obvious obstacles for synthesized learning connections that build on previous learning. Third, the disheartened morale and dissatisfaction of many nurses drains valuable energy and motivation integral to learning. Finally, the number of nurses formally prepared in transcultural nursing at the undergraduate or graduate level who are actively employed in an HCI and who can adeptly develop their own and others' cultural competence is grossly inadequate.

Although the removal of obstacles and challenges is one obvious solution, it is beyond the scope of this book to tackle these issues. The author contends that offering strategies and incentives for ongoing cultural competence development (part of professional development), combined with tangible patient, personal, and professional outcomes, will positively affect nurses' satisfaction and morale, thereby improving nurse retention and further enhancing patient care. Nurse educators, executives, and leaders in the HCI are empowered to make a tremendous difference by promoting, facilitating, and evaluating cultural competence development. Each individual nurse, nurse educator, executive, or leader is empowered to make a positive difference; however, the greatest impact will be achieved through a coordinated, holistic group effort that thoughtfully weaves together relevant high-priority educational programs, unit-based initiatives, and supplementary resources.

Certain factors within the HCI may support cultural competence development; yet, other factors may restrict its development. This chapter proposes some strategies for systematic inquiry into already existing facets of the HCI, while also suggesting strategies for developing new initiatives. This chapter aims to (a) uncover, discover, and explore educational opportunities (within HCIs) for promoting cultural competency; (b) describe action-focused strategies for educational innovation; and (c) present ideas for evaluation (and re-evaluation) of educational innovation implementation. Figures, tables, "Innovations in Cultural Competence Education" boxes, and the "Educator-In-Action" vignette provide supplementary information to expand on narrative text features. Major emphasis is placed on self-appraisal and determining educational priorities and goals.

SELF-ASSESSMENT

Similar to the process of cultural competency development in academia (see chapter 5), promoting cultural competency in the HCI requires considerable, sincere effort that must begin with self-assessment. Systematic self-assessment evaluates the various dimensions that can impact the educational process and the achievement of educational outcomes (Jeffreys, 2004). Figure 6.2 depicts a systematic assessment within the HCI setting. Here, self-assessment refers to assessment of the individual staff nurse, nurse manager, nurse educator, nurse executive, administrator, and the organization. (Readers are encouraged to refer to chapter 5 for in-depth discussion about self-assessment and Table 1.2 about dimensions of cultural values and beliefs [CVB]). Finally, self-assessment should conclude with a listing of strengths, weaknesses, gaps in knowledge, goals, commitment, desire, motivation, and priorities.

As mentioned in chapter 5, comprehensive understanding, skill, and desire are essential, but not enough to effectively make a positive difference in cultural competence development. The author believes that resilient transcultural self-efficacy (TSE) (confidence) is the integral component necessary in the process of cultural competence development (of self and in others). TSE is the mediating factor that enhances persistence in cultural competence development, despite obstacles, hardships, or stressors. Resilient TSE perceptions embrace lifelong learning in the quest to become "more" culturally competent and in the quest to assist others (learners) to become more culturally competent.

Within the HCI, there are many stressors or obstacles; therefore, it becomes increasingly important that individual staff nurses, nurse

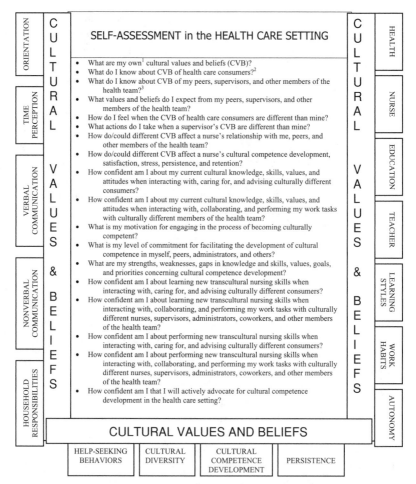

Figure 6.2 Self-assessment in the health care setting. [1]*Own* refers to individual staff nurses, nurse manager, executive, administrator, educator, or organization. [2]*Health care consumers* refer to individual patients, families, and communities. [3]*Other members of the health team* include professional and unlicensed health care providers. (Adapted from Jeffreys, M. R. (2004). *Nursing student retention: Understanding the process and making a difference.* New York, Springer p. 169. Used by permission, Springer Publishing Company, Inc., New York 10036).

managers, nurse educators, nurse executives, administrators, and the organization develop and maintain resilience, motivation, commitment, and persistence for endeavors that foster cultural competence. It is proposed that individuals (and the organization) with resilient TSE perceptions persist in their endeavors to be active transcultural advocates or promoters of

cultural competence in all dimensions of the HCI and professional practice. Table 6.1 provides a guide for appraising values, beliefs, and actions,
and for determining whether one is an active role model in cultural competence development within the HCI or whether there are factors restricting
cultural competence development. It is proposed that the "actions taken to
promote cultural competence development" is what makes one an active
role model. Active role models influence cultural competence development in others by presenting opportunities for vicarious learning and via
forms of persuasion (honest and judicious encouragement and feedback).
By providing ongoing opportunities for high-quality mentoring, HCI can
enhance the power of modeling on self-efficacy appraisal and development of nurses at all levels within the HCI. The power of mentoring on
nurses' professional development, satisfaction, quality of patient care, and
retention has been well documented (Cavanaugh & Huse, 2004; Heller,
Drenkard, Esposito-Herr, Romano, Tom, & Valentine, 2004; Vance &
Olson, 1998).

In addition, one must evaluate whether the HCI is truly committed
to the goal of cultural competence development and culturally congruent patient care for the right reasons. The right reasons mean guided by
altruism, ethics, and patient advocacy, rather than being motivated by
accrediting body criteria that mandate evidence of cultural competence
among employees and cultural competent health care among diverse client
populations. This needs to be considered because the relatively recent addition of cultural competence criteria by accrediting agencies correlates
with many HCI scrambling to produce evidence of cultural competence,
especially when cultural competence was previously invisible, superficial,
and/or unimportant. One approach is to examine whether the HCI actively embraced cultural diversity and had cultural competence as a goal
paired with opportunities for staff development prior to accrediting agencies' criteria mandating cultural competence. Actively embracing cultural
diversity includes multiple, intensive strategies designed to recruit, retain,
and encourage educational and career advancement among culturally diverse nurses, especially from groups underrepresented in nursing practice
and nursing leadership. Tragically, cultural diversity within the nursing
profession does not mirror the U.S. population; nurse leaders from underrepresented groups are even less visible (Burnes Bolton, 2004; Foley
& Wurmser, 2004; Georges, 2004; Simpson, 2004; Swanson, 2004; Villarruel & Peragallo, 2004; Washington, Erickson, & Ditomassi, 2004).
(The critical topic of enhancing cultural diversity within nursing is enormous; readers are referred to the current literature on nurse recruitment,
retention, and professional advancement.)

A second approach is to consider "If the accrediting agency re-
moved cultural competence from their evaluative criteria, would the HCI

Table 6.1   Self-Assessment: Active Promoter of Cultural Competence Development in the Health Care Institution

Promoter	Values, Beliefs, and Actions	Promoter
Yes	Views cultural competence as important in own[a] life *and shares beliefs with others*[b,c]	No
Yes	Views cultural competence as important in staff's education, professional development, and future practice *and shares view with others*	No
Yes	Views own role to include active involvement in promoting cultural competence development among staff members *and shares view with others*	No
Yes	Routinely updates own knowledge and skills to enhance cultural competence *and shares relevant information with others*	No
Yes	Attends professional events concerning cultural competence development *and shares positive and relevant experiences with others*	No
Yes	Views professional event participation concerning cultural competence development as important in staff members' ongoing continuing education, professional development, and future practice *and shares view with others*	No
Yes	*Offers incentives to encourage staff members' participation in professional events*	No
Yes	Maintains professional partnerships focused on cultural competence development *and shares positive and relevant experiences with others*	No
Yes	Maintains membership(s) in professional organizations whose primary mission is cultural competence development *and shares positive and relevant experiences with others*	No
Yes	Views memberships in professional organizations/associations (whose primary mission is cultural competence development) as important in staff's continuing education, professional development, and future practice *and shares view with others*	No
Yes	*Offers incentives to encourage others' participation in memberships in professional organizations/associations committed to cultural competence development*	No
Yes	Recognizes actual and potential barriers hindering the development of cultural competence *and initiates strategies to remove barriers*	No
Yes	*Implements strategies to encourage staff's development of cultural competence*	No
Yes	*Evaluates strategies implemented to encourage staff's development of cultural competence*	No

[a] *Own* refers to individual staff nurses, nurse manager, executive, administrator, educator, or organization.
[b] Active promoter/facilitator actions are indicated by *italics*.
[c] Other members of the health team include professional and unlicensed health care providers.
Adapted from Jeffreys, M. R. (2004). *Nursing student retention: Understanding the process and making a difference*. New York, Springer p. 191. Used by permission, Springer Publishing Company, Inc. New York 10036.

and its employees still allocate the same amount of time, money, and energy toward cultural competence development or would cultural competence be less valued?" These two major considerations are important because nurses exist within the organizational culture of HCI and are greatly influenced by the opportunities, values, and expectations provided by HCI (Thorpe & Loo, 2003). Organizational cultures truly committed to cultural competence exert positive influence on nurses' values, commitment, satisfaction, and motivation (Leininger, 1994b). Furthermore, organizations that actively reach out to culturally diverse patients, nurses, and communities provide a wealth of opportunities and benefits to all.

Motivation behind nurses' participation in cultural competence development in-services, continuing education, and/or workshops may not be optimal. For example, a nurse who attends a workshop because it is required for continued employment, salary increase, promotion, and/or transfer is extrinsically motivated by selfish, personal reasons rather than intrinsically motivated by altruism, the desire for professional and personal growth and development, and improved patient care. Consequently, multidimensional learner characteristics will need to be evaluated before the design of any educational interventions. Typically, educators within HCI are challenged with providing high-quality educational programs for nurses who represent cultural, educational, and career diversity (Bibb et al., 2003; Billings, 2004; Collins, 2002; Harrington & Walker, 2004; Mathews, 2003; Rashotte & Thomas, 2002). Developing strategies to shift extrinsic motivation to intrinsic motivation is one challenge for the HCI sincerely committed to developing cultural competence at high levels of excellence. The author contends that cultural competence is unachievable unless individuals are intrinsically motivated; resilient TSE (confidence) will positively influence intrinsic motivation and persistence at cultural competence development of self and others.

EVALUATION IN THE HEALTH CARE INSTITUTION

Following the template for systematic evaluation in the academic setting (see chapter 5), evaluation in the HCI begins with examining how visible (or invisible) cultural competency development is actively present (a) overall within the institution, (b) specifically at the individual unit (site) level, and (c) via outside connections to supplementary resources. A systematic evaluative inquiry should also be guided by two additional questions: (a) To what degree is cultural competence an integral component within the HCI? and (b) How do the cultural components

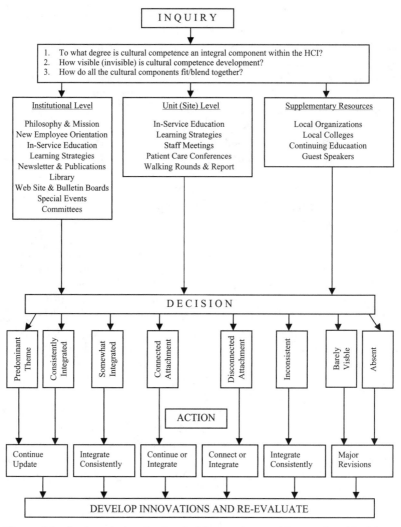

Figure 6.3 Systematic inquiry for decision, action, and innovation: Health care institutions (HCI).

fit together? (Figure 6.3) A thorough evaluation of what currently exists serves as a valuable precursor to informed decisions, responsible actions, and new diagnostic-prescriptive innovations targeting staff development and improved patient care outcomes. The following sections address major areas for inquiry, action, and innovation within the HCI.

Institution

Careful perusal of the HCI's philosophy, mission, and purpose may lend valuable insight into the HCI's worldview (perspective) on resources, resource allocation, profit goals, cultural diversity, cultural competence development, targeted patient populations and objectives, employee empowerment, nursing profession, decision making, and organizational priorities. For example, a nonprofit HCI whose mission statement and philosophy attest to provide culturally congruent health care to culturally diverse individuals, despite ability to pay, provides some beginning, favorable information concerning the desire to achieve cultural competence. However, without sufficient resources or strategies to (a) develop cultural competence of health care providers, (b) create cultural-specific professional care actions, and/or (c) evaluate strategy outcomes, positive goal achievement is unlikely. Close inspection at the institutional level must also assess whether cultural competency development is emphasized substantially, equally, and symmetrically throughout the HCI beyond philosophy, mission, and purpose to such areas as new employee orientation, in-service education, learning strategies, newsletters and publications, library, web site, bulletin boards, special events, and committees. Unfortunately, budget constraints, staffing shortage, and hospital restructuring has resulted in decreased HCI resources for new employee orientation, in-service education, and continuing education (Ellerton & Gregor, 2003; Pinkerton, 2004; Williams & Jones, 2004). Sample innovations particularly important to the development of cultural competence are presented in the Educator-in-Action vignette and can also be used to guide inquiry. Several major areas are described as follows.

New Employee Orientation

New employee orientation has the potential to initially introduce and reinforce the HCI's philosophy and purposes specifically concerning cultural competence development. Achievement of cultural competence must expand beyond meeting minimum levels of proficiency in clinical practice (product outcome view) to expecting ongoing efforts aimed at cultural competence development in self and others (process view). Nurse educators at new employee orientations have the potential to make a tremendous difference by introducing, emphasizing, fostering, and nurturing cultural competence development throughout the new employee orientation. Emphasizing ongoing education as a professional commitment to lifelong learning has the potential to raise motivation for learning. By presenting learning goals and outcomes with long-term broader professional and personal benefits rather than as merely employer expectations, occupational tasks, or job requirements, the emphasis will be on professional expectations, standards, and excellence. Emphasis on autonomy, accountability, self-regulation, and ethics is consistent with professional standards and expectations (ANA, 2001, 2003, 2004) and can serve as intrinsic motivators (Kubsch, Henniges, Lorenzoni, Eckardt, & Oleniczak, 2003). In contrast, mandatory workshops without connections to professionalism limit outcome results (Jones-Schenk & Yoder-Wise, 2002). Linking new employee learning with unit-specific examples and connections with other HCI resources and supplementary resources illustrates an easily accessible pathway to continue on the journey of cultural competence development paved by HCI's instrumental and philosophical support for cultural competence endeavors. For example, case study discussion and reflection transform passive classroom orientation into active, multidimensional, and synthesized learning (Rashotte & Thomas, 2002; Tomey, 2003; White, Amos, & Kouzekanani, 1999). Supplementing learning with CAI programs, web-based programs, satellite TV programs, videotapes, and simulation programs are other innovative options discussed in the literature (Bibb et al., 2002; Harrington & Walker, 2004; JCAHO, 2002; Mateo & McMyler, 2004; Matzo, Sherman, Mazanec, Barber, Virani, McLaughlin, 2002; Pastuszak & Rodowicz, 2002; Piercy, 2004; Squires, 2002).

As adult learners, new employees' motivation will be heightened with direct application and explicit ties to the unit (site) level. Partnering follow-up learning activities on the unit (site) level provides opportunities for applying general principles to specific patient situations. Assessing learner characteristics (including TSE perceptions) and pairing learners with experienced mentors who can serve as role models and offer encouragement will enhance cultural competence development. Self-efficacy perceptions will be greatly enhanced by role models who display effort and perform tasks successfully, rather than by role models who complete the task effortlessly (Bandura, 1986; Schunk, 1987).

Physiological indices such as manifestations of stress and anxiety also interfere with confidence and learning (Bandura, 1986). Typically, the stress of a new job, and perhaps a new career (for graduate nurses) exist during employee orientations, thereby creating additional challenges. Although nurse residency programs or postgraduate training programs for new graduate nurses may present positive solutions, financial constraints and scarce human resources present grave limitations (JCAHO, 2002). Sufficient supports for graduate nurses during the transitional process may include mentors, preceptors, prolonged general and unit-based orientation, review of reality shock phenomena and strategies for successful coping, positive professional socialization opportunities, and ongoing support beyond the orientation and probation period (Duchscher, 2004).

Unit (Site) Level

Although accountability for cultural competence development and culturally congruent health care delivery is a shared responsibility of individual staff nurses, nurse educators, and nurse managers, the nurse manager is ultimately responsible for holding staff accountable for developing and maintaining competencies (Mateo & McMyler, 2004). Delineating clear expectations and penalties for noncompliance, offering supportive strategies and rewards for developing competence, initiating corrective measures when necessary, and acknowledging positive achievements optimizes the occurrence of successful outcomes and minimizes the risk of noncompliance (Mateo & McMyler, 2004). Again, emphasizing the importance of cultural competence development as a lifelong commitment to professional development and the enhancement of patient care reminds nurses of their individual responsibility to uphold professional standards. Thus, the shifted emphasis on individual professional accountability attempts to stimulate and nurture intrinsic motivation, thereby replacing the potentially previously held, predominant influence of extrinsic motivators with true motivation and commitment.

Objectively appraising the daily routines, rituals, and activities specific within the unit (setting) and within the context of cultural competence and culturally congruent patient care as desirable outcomes requires time, expertise, and dedication. Table 6.2 presents select activities with cultural competence application common across a variety of settings. Because culturally congruent patient care begins with accurate, sensitive assessment of individual patient's cultural values, beliefs, practices, and behaviors, it is essential that the initial health history interview and physical examination incorporate cultural components visibly and substantially. Inspection of the demographic form and health history interview (institution or unit specific) should be free of bias and reflect key cultural assessment areas particularly relevant for the setting or unit. For example, are patients (a) invited to self-identify with ethnic group affiliation(s) as an open-ended question; (b) asked to select one or more ethnic group affiliation options, including an open-ended fill-in; (c) instructed to pick one category only; or (d) assigned a category by the admission nurse or physician? Examining whether health history forms include details about folk medicine practices, home remedies, spiritual rituals, and non-Western health practices should also appraise whether questions are presented equally with questions about Western medicine and whether questions are presented first, last, integrated, or as an afterthought. Subtle, culturally incongruent, and insensitive messages may often be unintentional or unconsciously incompetent; however, they can hinder communication and assessment. Second, information forms are only meaningful if nurses (and other health

Table 6.2   Select Activities With Cultural Competence Application

Activity	Cultural competence application
Health history interview	• Systematic cultural assessment incorporated within the health history interview • Interview form reflects key cultural assessment areas particularly relevant for setting or unit
Physical exam	• Physical exam assessments and documentation are adapted to meet cultural needs and biophysical differences • Physical exam form is free of cultural biases and includes physical assessment areas particularly relevant for setting or unit and for numerous different cultural groups
Change of shift report	Cultural specific care actions (Leininger, 1991a) are discussed: • Preservation or maintenance • Accommodation or negotiation • Repatterning or restructuring
Patient record	Cultural-specific care actions (Leininger, 1991a) are documented: • Preservation or maintenance • Accommodation or negotiation • Repatterning or restructuring
Patient care plan Patient teaching plan Patient discharge plan	Cultural specific care actions (Leininger, 1991a) are planned, implemented, and evaluated: • Preservation or maintenance • Accommodation or negotiation • Repatterning or restructuring
Patient care conferences	• Topics focus on cultural competence development • Clinical topics include relevant case exemplars representing culturally diverse patients
Walking rounds	Incorporate culturally congruent approaches for introductions, communication, and physical exam
Staff meetings	• Incorporate culturally appropriate strategies for cultural diverse staff • Address issues and topics to enhance cultural competence • Promote multicultural workplace harmony • Promote culturally congruent patient care • Include resources with cultural expertise as needed
Multidisciplinary communication and collaboration	Incorporate culturally congruent approaches for introductions, communication, and designing cultural specific care actions
Unit-based in-service education	• Topics focus on cultural competence development • Clinical topics include relevant case exemplars representing culturally diverse patients • Use multidimensional teaching–learning strategies that incorporate cognitive, practical, affective dimensions, and transcultural self-efficacy • Relevant journal articles and other resources are available • Relevant information is posted on staff bulletin board or in communication book
Patient teaching materials	Include literature and resources specific to consumer's ethnicity, religion, preferred language, socioeconomic status, geographic location, developmental level, educational level, and health needs

professionals) have the appropriate knowledge, skills, values, and confidence to use them appropriately with culturally diverse patients and to document findings clearly.

It is important that assessment findings be translated into cultural specific and congruent plans of care; however, this activity must extend beyond mere written documentation. Active integration of culturally congruent patient care must extend throughout all unit (setting)-based activities such as change of shift report, walking rounds, patient care conferences, patient teaching, delegation of tasks, staff meetings, and multidisciplinary collaboration. Realistic and feasible opportunities for ongoing staff development and in-service education are enhanced through multidimensional teaching–learning innovations. Especially in times of limited financial and human resources, it is essential to determine priorities based on immediate needs, learner characteristics, and available resources.

PRIORITIZATION

Following transcultural generalist principles introduced or reintroduced at new employee orientation and reinforced through later in-services, subsequent educational opportunities for cultural competence development should be available, building on previous knowledge, skills, values, and confidence. Promoting cultural competence is a broad, massive topic to undertake, therefore determining which priority focus areas will assist in the justification for allocation of limited resources (e.g., time, money, expertise). The first question "What are the priority issues or focus areas?" is subsequently followed by the second question "How can priority issues be determined?" Although several approaches may be employed, this chapter presents a strategy comprised of three main considerations: (a) target populations, (b) learner characteristics, and (c) educational resources. Table 6.3 presents sample questions to guide prioritization.

Determining target patient populations may be initiated throughout the HCI with specific focus on select units or be initiated at the unit-based level. The method of determining patient target areas should first begin by determining the presence of cultural groups present within the geographic region. Then, which groups use, do not use, or underuse health care services should be determined, thereby contrasting actual patient profiles with potential patient profiles. Decisions can be further guided by considering national goals in eliminating health disparities and local issues. Justifiable and feasible rationale for the selected group must be defensible when considering learner characteristics and educational resources. In other words, target population selection should not be determined in isolation from other major considerations (see Box 6.4, Educator-in-Action Vignette). Detailing an initial broad list of potential target patient populations demonstrates the existence of diverse cultural groups typically grouped together under broad demographic categories. If health care is to be truly culturally congruent, then culture care must be specific to each cultural group, necessitating differentiation within and between groups. Figure 6.4 presents a sample broad and detailed list.

Table 6.3 Sample Questions to Guide Prioritization

Target Populations

1. Which cultural groups are present in the geographic region and *use* health care services?
2. Which cultural groups are present in the geographic region and *do not use* or *underuse* health care services?
3. Of these groups, which ones should be targeted first?
4. Why? What is the underlying rationale?
   • Significant health problem
   • Largest cultural group
   • Newest cultural group
   • Victims of discrimination and bias
   • Marginalized group
   • Group poorly understood by health care personnel
   • Other
5. What are the specific desired goals for the targeted population(s)?

Learner Characteristics

1. What are learners' background, identity, values, and beliefs?

Profile Characteristics	*Affective Factors*
Age	Cultural values and beliefs
Ethnicity	Transcultural self-efficacy
Race	Motivation
Gender	
Socioeconomic	
Religion	
Primary (first) language	
Prior education	
Prior work experience	

2. What are learner strengths?
3. What are learner weaknesses?
4. What learning gaps are/may be present?
5. What biases are/may be present?
6. What prior *formalized* learning (related to culture) can provide a foundation for continued and ongoing learning?

Educational Resources

1. What learning opportunities for transcultural nursing exist(ed)?
2. What are the specific desired goals for the targeted population(s)?
3. What resources are currently available?
4. What resources are necessary to achieve goals of developing cultural competency for targeted population(s)?
5. What resources are most easily attainable?
6. Who can design, implement, and evaluate multidimensional strategies to maximize learning?

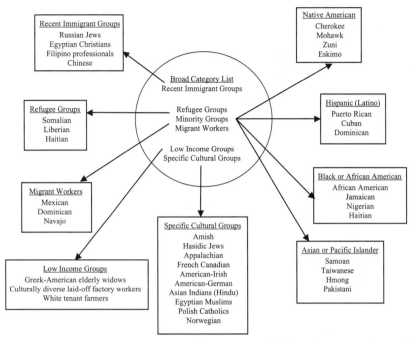

Figure 6.4 Determining target populations—sample broad category list and sample detailed list.

A decision based on comprehensive assessment of patient populations, learner characteristics, and educational resources proposes realistic goals capitalizing on learner strengths and educational resources. Furthermore, creatively designing multidimensional teaching–learning activities to enhance cultural competence development has the potential to bring learning to higher levels of synthesis and internalization and foster realistic self-efficacy appraisal and resilience. Ongoing in-service education or a series of transcultural workshops are two examples of education initiatives coordinated through staff development. Although this is important, fragmented educational components that are (or seem) disconnected from each other and from other activities within the HCI offer limited opportunities for cultural competence development. Coordinating the development of cognitive, practical, and affective learning requires much planning and interconnectedness. Connecting innovations in cultural competence education may be achieved through publicity, publications, special events, and committees and by developing a collaborative network of supplementary resources beyond the HCI. For example, if the systematic decision-making process results in the decision to target "Enhancing

Cultural Competence in the Care of Recent Egyptian Immigrants," connecting innovations may be done by performing the following:

- Publicizing workshop series on bulletin boards, staff web site or listserv, hospital Internet site, staff meeting announcement, flyer attached to paycheck, personal letter, flyers, personal communication between unit liaison nurse on each shift who will personally invite other staff nurses, hospital newsletter, and/or local newspaper and TV announcements.
- Purchasing, borrowing, organizing, and displaying relevant professional and consumer literature in HCI library.
- Offering traditional Egyptian food choices every Thursday for 2 months in the cafeteria, partnered with posters and handouts describing the food choices, cultural meaning of food, nutritional values, method of preparation, estimated cost per serving, dietary accommodations for patients on specific prescribed diets, and other relevant information. (Avoid planning activity during months with large number of religious fast days.)
- Featured cultural expert who will participate in the workshop series, continuing education program, consultation, and/or conference.
- Relevant journal article, brief article summary outline, appropriate referral resources, and pertinence to specific unit posted on staff bulletin boards on each unit.
- Agenda for the monthly institutional committee meeting for cultural competence development focuses on designated topic.
- Collaboration and cosponsorship of conference focused on (or incorporating) selected topic with relevant Ethnic Nursing Association, local chapter of Transcultural Nursing Society, or other professional association.
- Creating an advisory board focused on selected topic with related local organizations, universities, community groups, staff nurses, nurse educators, nurse executives, and other members of the multidisciplinary health care team.
- Quality assurance team develops comprehensive plan to evaluate educational innovations.

EVALUATION

The most comprehensive education evaluation plan includes formative and summative components that are explicitly tied to the educational strategy's goal and purpose and are objectively measured. Formative evaluations assess the process of a strategy rather than outcomes and can be monitored as the strategy is implemented. Through systematic and ongoing formative evaluations, the documentation of specific activities and the identification of desired outcomes and anticipated strengths, as well as any difficulties, snags, weaknesses, and/or problems, will allow for diagnostic-prescriptive modifications based on learner's feedback obtained from consistent qualitative and quantitative data collection. Summative evaluations assess the achievement of desired learning outcomes or program outcomes and are monitored at the completion of the teaching strategy or educational program. Summative evaluations are strengthened via a multidimensional approach that includes cognitive, practical, and affective components using quantitative and qualitative data.

Every educational evaluation plan should include formative and evaluative components that are realistic, positively phrased, and provide valid, valuable feedback. Evaluation plans that are unrealistic and difficult to measure objectively should be avoided because data will be invalid, unreliable, and therefore useless. For example, a formative evaluation goal that states "All cultural competence workshop participants will rate all speakers as 'excellent'" does not allow for disparate responses that discriminate between different speakers' strengths. Disparate and discriminating responses are desirable to substantiate validity of responses or respondents' ability and willingness to think carefully about each item, differentiate between items, and select a thoughtful and honest response (Sudman & Bradburn, 1991). Modification of this goal as "The majority (or 80%) of cultural competence workshop participants will be satisfied with the overall program and individual program components as seen by at least 80% of workshop participants selecting a "4 – satisfied" or "5 – very satisfied" on the Workshop Evaluation Survey Tool (WEST). Box 6.1 presents an example of a formative evaluation plan, data collection, data analysis, and future implications. This example could be adapted to evaluate other cultural competence education initiatives within the institution, unit (setting) level, and supplementary (collaborative) resources.

Box 6.1   Innovations in cultural competence education: Formative evaluation plan, implementation, and implications

Goal: Staff nurses are satisfied with the Cultural Competence Development Series workshops as seen by 80% of nurses selecting "4" (satisfied) or "5" (very satisfied) on the Workshop Evaluation Survey Tool (WEST).

Data Collection: WEST is administered after workshop 1 in a series of five planned "Enhance Your Cultural Competency" workshops given during the next 12 months.

Quantitative Data Analysis indicates

- Overall satisfaction
- Eighty-seven percent of nurses selected "4" or "5" responses on the majority of WEST items
- Ninety-two percent of nurses selected "4" or "5" responses on items concerning satisfaction with learning outcomes achieved within cognitive, practical, and affective domains
- High satisfaction with speaker 1 and with the video
- Moderate satisfaction with guest speaker 2 and with the PowerPoint slides

Qualitative Data: Comments from respondents suggest that

- Speaker 2 should wear a microphone and slides should be larger
- Workshops should be 15 minutes longer to allow for questions and to enhance learning
- Participants were unaware of the impact of their own CVB on the care of culturally different patients
- Workshop participants expressed appreciation at being asked for their feedback

Empirically Based Interventions for Quality Improvement (some possibilities):

- Continue with workshop series
- Invite speaker 1 back and continue to show the video
- Invite speaker 2 back, provided he or she uses a microphone and revises (enlarges) slides*
- Extend workshops 15 minutes to allow for questions and dialog*
- Provide opportunity for nurses to discuss and share their raised awareness with each other*
- Continue to administer WEST after each workshop, and modify or continue with educational strategies
- Continue to emphasize importance of participants' feedback*

---

*Rationale for these interventions was provided by the solicitation of qualitative comments. Making decisions based solely on quantitative data is self-limiting. For example, based solely on the quantitative data in this scenario, speaker 2 might not have been invited back as a presenter, despite his or her expertise.

Within the HCI, summative evaluations may often target both measurable changes in the learner and changes in patient outcomes. If changes are to be truly documented, it is extremely important that pretest measures are conducted before any strategy is implemented and that strategies are followed by appropriate posttest measures that permit valid and reliable data analyses. Without pre- and posttests, the influence of the intervention on the dependent variable(s) cannot be established. Although qualitative methodologies provide unique, valuable data that are usually otherwise unobtainable, the reality of current funding initiatives is that strong quantitative findings generally substantiate further funding for teaching and practice innovations. Qualitative data will add richness to the overall understanding of the phenomenon under investigation, thereby providing valuable information to guide future strategy interventions.

Constraints in HCI resources (e.g., money, staff, time, equipment) place increasing demands on conserving resources to those endeavors that have proved positive, desirable outcomes. "The return on investment in nursing will be reflected both in cost savings and in improvements in the safety and quality of care provided" (JCAHO, 2002, p. 17). It is therefore beneficial and essential to have patient outcome indicators that increase HCI revenue, income, or access; decrease costs; or other positive outcomes. Such outcome measures necessitate quantitative methodology (see Box 6.2). Unfortunately, few studies have investigated the impact of cultural competence education on health outcomes, patient behavior change, satisfaction, or health care delivery (Fortier & Bishop, 2003), although the impact of culturally congruent patient care on clinical outcomes has been demonstrated (Management Sciences for Health [MSH], 2005). Measurable outcome indicators are needed (OMH, 2005). Cost savings can be demonstrated with increased nurse retention, increased staffing that eliminates the need for overtime or outside agency nurses, decreased staffing vacancies, and/or decreased absences that are specifically correlated with increased nurses' satisfaction following a sequence of workshops, special events, or other cultural competence initiatives. Evaluating changes in learners' TSE perceptions using the Transcultural Self-Efficacy Tool (TSET) presents a quantitative measure for evaluating changes within cognitive, practical, and affective dimensions (see Box 6.3).

Box 6.2   Innovations in cultural competence education: Summative evaluation—sample for measuring changes in patient outcomes (access, quality, and cost)

Desired Outcome 1: Patient satisfaction among Mexican American patients at the diabetic outpatient clinic will increase following diabetic clinic registered nurses' completion of five Culturally Congruent Care for Mexican Americans workshops and as measured by the Patient Satisfaction Survey (PSS).

- *Data Collection:* Administer PSS to Mexican American patients at the diabetic clinic before the start of workshop 1 and 1 month after workshop 5 (cross-sectional study design).
- *Data Analysis:* Compare survey results.
  - *Quantitative:*
    - Did PSS scores change in the expected direction?
    - What were patients most satisfied about?

- What were patients least satisfied about?
- Would patients refer others to use general hospital services?
- *Qualitative:* What comments and common themes emerged?

Desired Outcome 2: Hospitalization rates and emergency room usage among Mexican American diabetic clinic patients will decrease and regularly scheduled attendance at diabetic clinic appointments will increase following registered nurse completion of workshop 5 (increased access to primary preventive care, increased quality, decreased cost).

- *Data Collection:* Collect relevant data monthly for 3 months before initiating workshop 1, monthly during workshop series, and then monthly for 6 months after workshop 5. (Also, collect other data such as staffing trends, workshop series participants, and nurse retention to check for control, consistency, and/or extraneous variables.)
- *Data Analysis:* Compare rates.
  - What data trends occurred?
  - What were the statistically significant results?
  - Were there any threats to internal and external validity?

Desired Outcome 3: Hospital revenue will increase as seen by increased number of new patients (using any hospital services) referred by Mexican American patients attending the diabetic clinic, by hearing about hospital's Culturally Congruent Care for Mexican Americans staff workshops, or by hearing about cultural sensitivity of nurses.

- *Data Collection:* Four months before initiating workshops and then monthly for 1 year after workshop 1 is initiated, survey new patients (using any hospital services) about why they chose hospital.
- *Data Analysis:* Calculate number of new patients and hospital revenue generated from new patients who chose hospital services based on previous three criteria. Compare and contrast data.

Desired Outcome 4: Hospital profits will exceed losses as seen by higher income generated from increased use of diabetic clinic services among Mexican Americans and decreased losses incurred from unpaid hospital costs resulting from managed care reimbursement guidelines.

- *Data Collection:* Collect respective data following method described in Desired Outcome 2.
- *Data Analysis:* Analyze respective data following method described in Desired Outcome 2.

---

*Rationale for these interventions was provided by the solicitation of qualitative comments. Making decisions based solely on quantitative data is self-limiting. For example, based solely on the quantitative data in this scenario, speaker 2 might not have been invited back as a presenter, despite his or her expertise.

Box 6.3   Innovations in cultural competence education:
Summative evaluation—changes in transcultural
self-efficacy perceptions with implications

Goal: Workshop participants will demonstrate positive changes in cultural competence development as seen by changes in subscale mean scores on the TSET in the anticipated direction from pretest to posttest.

Data Collection: TSET is administered before Enhance Your Cultural Competency workshop 1 and after the last (fifth) workshop.

Data Analysis:
Calculations on TSET pretest and TSET posttest

- SEST scores (mean) were calculated for each subscale.
- Unable to perform factor analysis because current sample size was too small; therefore, factors derived in Jeffreys and Smodlaka (1998) study were used to calculate mean scores for each factor.
- It was an underlying assumption that no nurses in this setting would select "1" or "2" responses on 20% or more of subscale responses; therefore, SEL was not calculated.
- Nurses were divided into low, medium, and high groups for each subscale using the "+1/−1 standard deviation from the mean" methodology.
- To determine items that nurses were most or least confident about in each dimension, item means for the group were rank ordered within each subscale.

Comparative Tests:

- To detect significant differences between pretests and posttests on all calculations listed previously, *t* tests were performed.

Results (select examples):

- On both pretests and posttests, nurses were least confident with their knowledge and most confident about their values, attitudes, and beliefs concerning culturally different clients.
- Overall, nurses had statistically significant changes (increase) in SEST scores from pretest to posttest on the Cognitive and Practical subscales.
- Statistically significant changes were not detected on the Affective Subscale, although scores changed in the anticipated direction (increase).
- Statistically significant changes occurred for each of the factors, except "self-awareness."
- For each subscale, nurses in the "low" group on pretest demonstrated the greatest change in self-efficacy perceptions on the posttest.
- Demographic data indicated that the majority of nurses in the pretest "high" group on the Cognitive and Practical subscales and who remained in the posttest "high" group for these two subscales had

attended at least two conferences on cultural issues and/or completed a graduate course in transcultural nursing prior to the HCI workshop series.

Limitations: Sample size, other potential threats to internal and/or external validity

Interpretation (select examples):

- When examining the results in relation to underlying conceptual framework (CCC model), the results make sense conceptually.
- Statistically and practically significant changes occurred in anticipated directions (according to underlying conceptual framework and previous empirical results obtained using TSET). Therefore, the educational intervention made a measurable, significant difference in nurses' TSE perceptions.

Implications (some possibilities):

- Continue with cultural competence workshops and re-evaluate.
- Expand cultural competence workshops to target other settings within the HCI and re-evaluate.
- Expand cultural competence workshops to target physicians within the HCI and re-evaluate using TSET physician format.
- Target future cultural competence workshops to address items that nurses were least confident about and re-evaluate.

Preparation of a comprehensive summary report that substantially details and succinctly highlights key findings via tables, figures, and/or bulleted lists should be accompanied by easy-to-read descriptive text. A thorough, user-friendly evaluation that aims to include nurses (and multidisciplinary health care professionals) of varying levels of education and research expertise will enhance the application of the evaluation results and help prevent feelings of exclusion or being overwhelmed. The true potential of cultural competence development within the HCI can only be optimally realized when feelings of mutual respect, validation, inclusiveness, and group solidarity predominate, acknowledging the many important contributions each individual can make in promoting culturally congruent care. Creatively connecting the positive attributes and strengths of individuals within HCI will maximize the overall institution's positive outcomes related to cultural competence educational strategies and innovations.

KEY POINT SUMMARY

- The health care institution (HCI) assumes a great responsibility for assuring the public that nurses are prepared to provide culturally congruent care and that the care is appropriately rendered.
- Each individual nurse, nurse educator, executive, or leader is empowered to make a positive difference in cultural competence; however, the greatest impact will be achieved through a coordinated, holistic group effort that thoughtfully weaves together relevant high-priority educational programs, unit-based initiatives, and supplementary resources.
- Promoting cultural competency in the HCI requires considerable, sincere effort that must begin with self-assessment of the individual staff nurse, nurse manager, nurse educator, nurse executive, administrator, and organization.
- It is proposed that individuals (and the organization) with resilient transcultural self-efficacy (TSE) perceptions (confidence) persist in their endeavors to be active transcultural advocates or promoters of cultural competence in all dimensions of the HCI and professional practice.
- Cultural competence is unachievable unless individuals are intrinsically motivated; resilient TSE (confidence) will positively influence intrinsic motivation and persistence at cultural competence development of self and others.
- Selection of targeted priority areas should be based on a comprehensive assessment of patient populations, learner characteristics, and educational resources.
- Close inspection at the institutional level must assess whether cultural competency development is emphasized substantially, equally, and symmetrically throughout the HCI, beyond philosophy, mission, and purpose to such areas as new employee orientation, in-service education, learning strategies, newsletters and publications, library, web site, bulletin boards, special events, and committees.
- Connecting innovations in cultural competence education may be achieved through publicity, publications, special events, and committees, and by developing a collaborative network of supplementary resources beyond the HCI.
- Educational innovations should include a comprehensive formative and summative evaluation plan that is realistic, positively phrased, and measurable.

- Within the HCI, summative evaluations may often target both measurable changes in the learner and changes in patient outcomes.
- Evaluating changes in learners' TSE perceptions using the Transcultural Self-Efficacy Tool (TSET) presents a quantitative measure for evaluating changes within cognitive, practical, and affective dimensions.
- The true potential of cultural competence development within the HCI can only be optimally realized when feelings of mutual respect, validation, inclusiveness, and group solidarity predominate, acknowledging the many important contributions each individual can make in promoting culturally congruent care.

Box 6.4   Educator-in-Action Vignette

During a staff meeting, several staff nurses verbalize feelings of inadequacy and lower confidence when caring for new groups of immigrant populations. The nurses represent diversity in age, gender, education, ethnicity, religion, race, and number of years in nursing.

Stella, the nurse manager, recognizes the need to promote cultural competence development for care of patients of diverse cultures. She is also aware of the immediate priority to focus on select target groups, provide immediate feedback to these adult learners, and capitalize on learners' intrinsic motivation. Through guided questioning and dialog, Stella assists the staff nurses in determining populations within the broad category of "recent immigrants" by detailing subcategories. Three major recent immigrant groups are identified: Russian Jews, Filipinos, and Dominicans.

To determine which group should be targeted first, Stella uses the sample questions to guide target population prioritization (see Table 6.3). By writing nurses' rationale, concerns, and goals on the chalkboard, they can easily visualize differences and similarities between the three groups. For example, although each group consisted of non-English-speaking individuals, more Filipino clients were able to speak English than the other groups. Of the three groups, Dominicans sought primary care less frequently, often first entering the hospital system with acute illness, advanced illnesses, or complications from chronic illnesses. As a result, poorer health outcomes and prolonged hospitalization within the constraints of managed care reimbursement also presented the HCI with financial losses.

Ed, the unit's professional development specialist (nurse educator), invites nurses to share learner characteristics by asking them to write down on an index card information about prior formalized learning (related to culture), including continuing education programs and academic courses. Nurses are invited to share any other concerns, interests, or information that they think may be helpful in assisting with the decision and design of cultural competence development unit initiative. Here are some excerpts:

Maureen: "I graduated 2 years ago from a baccalaureate nursing program that had a required course in transcultural nursing. Culture care was integrated throughout my program, and I had many guided opportunities in clinical with culturally diverse patients. During my senior semester break, I participated in a volunteer health service initiative with the university, providing care for indigent patients in the Dominican Republic. That experience made me realize that I have a lot to learn about cultures that are different than mine. Some of the other staff nurses expect me to be the expert on Dominicans, but I am not confident about my knowledge and communication skills."

Rosa: "Because I speak Spanish fluently, many of the other nurses automatically think I know everything about the Dominican culture and customs. Of course, I can translate information, but sometimes I feel as though the patients and families are hesitant to trust me completely because I am not Dominican. It bothers me when my colleagues discount my concerns. One other nurse even said, 'It's all the same—Puerto Rican, Dominican, Cuban—you all speak Spanish.' That really hurt my feelings."

Svetlana: "I am not confident about dealing with so many of the different cultures in the United States. Although I got my associate degree in nursing last June and am attending school part time for my bachelor's degree, I still am overwhelmed by the differences from Russia where I spent 40 years of my life. I am proud to be a resource for the other nurses to help translate and provide quality care for the Russian patients."

Taylor: "I have attended several conferences on cultural competence presented by the state nurses' association and the National Black Nurses Association. Next June, I will be finished with my master's degree program. I think I would like to become an adjunct instructor at the university or a nurse educator within this institution, but I'm not sure. I feel it is important to have general background information about caring competently for cultures different than one's own. I would benefit from review of this necessary information first before focusing on any specific group."

Based on this information, Ed and Stella collaborate about learner strengths, weaknesses, learning gaps, biases, motivation, and confidence. Next, exploration of educational resources within the HCI reveals that an advanced practice nurse in the adult day hospital is also certified in transcultural nursing. Further exploration reveals that two nursing faculty members at a collaborating nearby university are actively involved in cultural competence research and teaching. Unfortunately, no one is a specialist within any of the three potential target populations; however, through professional associations and networks, an appropriate consultant/guest speaker could be selected.

Resource allocation (time, honorarium for consultant) for cultural competence program development, implementation, and evaluation is approved at all executive levels within the HCI. Results from the pilot initiative will serve to guide future educational endeavors. Changes in learners, patient outcomes, satisfaction, nursing staffing patterns, and costs will be evaluated.

Based on the assessment of target populations, learner characteristics, and educational resources, Ed, Stella, and the unit staff mutually agree to first focus on culturally congruent care for Dominican adults. This will occur only after introducing (or reviewing) general principles, skills, knowledge, concepts, and values concerning cultural competence (generalist approach).

Staff's survey results of preferred learning strategies support the use of the following innovative strategies:

- 15-minute PowerPoint presentation reviewing general principles of cultural competence development
  - Presentation by nurse educator or certified transcultural nurse (CTN) on each shift (weeks 1 and 2)
  - Posting of PowerPoint presentation on internal web site
  - Slide handouts posted on unit bulletin boards
  - Bibliography list with select articles and books available on unit
- Three journal articles on cultural competence and assessment (general) (weeks 2–4)
  - Posted on staff bulletin boards, internal web site, and unit staff listserv
  - Bullet list outlining 10 key points of article posted on staff bulletin board
  - Bag lunch (breakfast or dinner) discussion
- Three journal articles or book chapters on culturally congruent care for Dominican Americans (weeks 5–7)
  - (as above)
- Learning lunch with guest presenter/consultant (week 8)
  - Traditional Dominican foods prepared by Dominican American caterers
  - Cultural learning menu—one-paragraph description of food, meaning of food, etc.
  - 20-minute presentation
  - 15-minute group discussion
  - Edited video clip of presentation, foods, and discussion (with permission) on internal web site
- Weekly "tidbits and niblets" program (Williams & Jones, 2004) (weeks 9–13)
  - Tiny bytes of cultural information, questions, and answers with references on index cards
  - Contact hours awarded for each tidbit completed
- Exploring cultural resource links for professional education (week 10)
  - 15-minute presentation by librarian with appropriate expertise
  - Edited video clip and/or PowerPoint presentation on internal web site
- Learning breakfast with guest presenter/consultant (week 11)
  - (as above with learning lunch but different topic within same cultural group)
- Exploring cultural resource links for patient education (week 12)
  - 15-minute presentation by librarian with appropriate expertise

- Edited video clip and/or PowerPoint presentation on internal web site
- Learning dinner with guest presenter/consultant (week 13)
  - (as above with learning lunch but different topic within same cultural group)
- Panel discussion cosponsored by HCI, nearby university, and two local nursing associations (week 14)
- Staff meeting, discussion, and future plans (week 15)

CHAPTER 7

Professional Associations

Professional associations (see Figure 7.1) provide unique opportunities for professional socialization, networking, skill enhancement, knowledge expansion, and professional attitude development (Betts & Cherry, 2002; Joel & Kelly, 2002). Because professional associations possess a potentially powerful and extensive ability to network diverse and talented groups of professionals beyond a single health care institution (HCI) or academic setting, professional associations can exert tremendous influence on promoting, disseminating, and advancing cultural competence development. Collectively and individually, professional associations, leaders, and members are challenged to take definitive actions that prioritize and enhance cultural competence development. Each individual member is empowered to make a positive difference; however, the greatest impact will be achieved through a coordinated, holistic group effort that purposely interconnects all dimensions of the association. Although concentrated efforts and actions must occur on varying levels within the association, actions must also create a positive effect well beyond the association membership. Such actions necessitate empirically and conceptually supported inquiries, actions, and innovations motivated by true commitment for cultural competence that is reflected substantially in the professional association's philosophy and mission, structure, events, activities, and networks.

Despite the type of professional association (broad purpose association, specialty practice association, or special interest association), all professional associations have the potential to make a real difference in the cultural competence development of nurses and other health professionals and to enhance quality of care among culturally diverse patients. Certain factors within the professional association may support cultural competence development; yet, other factors may restrict its development. This chapter highlights strategies for (a) identifying educational

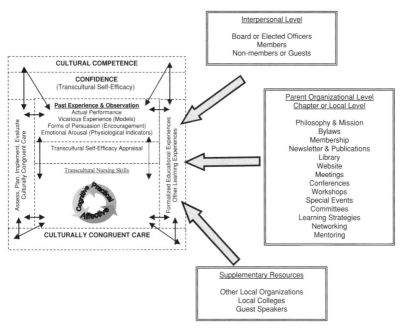

Figure 7.1 Professional associations.

opportunities (within professional associations) for promoting cultural competency, (b) recognizing and overcoming barriers and challenges, and (c) developing action-focused strategies for educational innovation. The following section addresses key features for inquiry, action, and educational innovation within the professional association.

EVALUATION IN THE PROFESSIONAL ASSOCIATION

Consistent with the evaluation of educational opportunities for cultural competence development in academic and health care settings, it is equally necessary to closely examine how visible (or invisible) cultural competency development is in the professional association. Within the professional association, examination of interpersonal characteristics, parent association and affiliated chapters, and supplementary resources requires courage, commitment, time, energy, and a systematic plan. A systematic evaluative inquiry can be guided by two additional questions: (a) To what degree is cultural competence an integral component? and (b) How do the dimensions of the association fit together to support cultural competence development? (see Figure 7.2). A thorough evaluation serves as a valuable precursor to informed decisions, responsible actions, and new innovations.

A detailed critique of the association's philosophy and mission, bylaws, membership, newsletter and publications, library, web site,

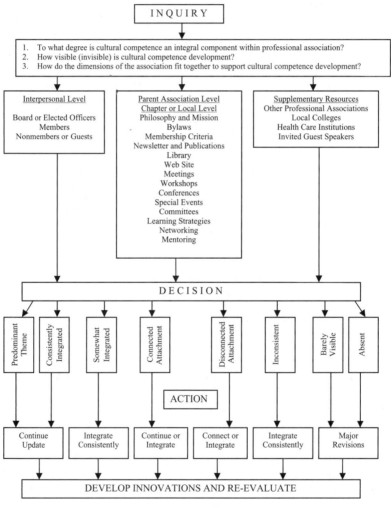

Figure 7.2 Systematic inquiry for decision, action, and innovation in professional associations.

meetings, workshops, conferences, special events, committees, learning strategies, networking, and mentoring is an ambitious endeavor, requiring much diligence, humility, honesty, and dedication. It may be a startling realization that a professional association is not as involved in cultural competence development as it could be (or should be). Systematic evaluation helps identify association strengths, weaknesses, inconsistencies, and gaps related to cultural competency development. Guided and purposeful reflective self-appraisal at an individual member level, parent association level, and/or chapter level will provide valuable insight and perspective. On close scrutiny, threads of culture and cultural competency should be equally and substantially evident throughout the association's structure, activities, and resources.

Examination must differentiate between superficial and substantial evidence. For example, a professional association may sponsor a workshop on "Health Promotion and African American Populations in Urban Communities," appearing to meet an association mission statement to "disseminate information to promote health among culturally diverse populations." Yet, the workshop may not actually promote cultural competence development if the multidimensional cultural values and beliefs (CVB) of a clearly defined cultural group are never thoroughly explored (see Table 7.1) As a second example, mission statements that incorporate such phrases as "cultural competence," "cultural diversity," and "culturally congruent care" may appear to value cultural competence. However, without the implementation of any actions and innovations that actively enhance cultural competence development, such mission statements are meaningless, misleading, and even harmful. Associations are challenged to effectively integrate cultural competence throughout all aspects of the association to provide long-lasting learning and desirable outcomes among culturally diverse professionals and beyond the immediate membership population. Because culturally diverse individuals have diverse learning needs, strengths, values, and beliefs, offering different types of multidimensional active learning activities will be most beneficial (Brookfield, 1986; Gaffney, 2000; Kelly, 1997; Williams & Calvillo, 2002; Yoder, 2001). (Various learning strategies are discussed in chapter 5.)

Close scrutiny of association brochures, membership applications, newsletters, journals, other publications, library, and web site should assess whether cultural competency development is emphasized substantially, equally, and symmetrically in all dimensions. Using the general questions depicted in Figure 7.2, associations can conduct a systematic inquiry, make a decision, choose an action, and then develop innovations. For example, if the consensus of the association's board members decide that cultural issues are "barely visible" in the association newsletter and web site, the action chosen should be to make major revisions, develop

Table 7.1 Going Beyond Topic and Title: Searching for Substantive Evidence of Cultural Competence

Topic/Title	Poor Example	Better Example
Prostate cancer (PC) screening practices among middle-age, African American (AA) men	1) Focuses on disease process and reported statistics of PC screening practices among AA men 2) Mortality rates correlated with late screening practices 3) Includes recent immigrants and/or refugees from Haiti, Trinidad, Jamaica, Barbados, Nigeria, Kenya, and South Africa, as well as descendents of American slaves	1) Introductory focus on cultural values and beliefs (CVB), as well as practices associated with health promotion and illness prevention 2) Specific focus on CVB, and practices associated with prostate screening among AA 3) Sample excludes immigrants, only including individuals descended from Africans brought to America as slaves and who self-identify as AA.
Culture and sensitivity for wound care—new innovations in clinical practice	Focuses on the diagnostic procedure of obtaining a wound culture, providing wound care, evaluating culture and sensitivity results, administering appropriate anti-infective medications, and evaluating healing	Presents an overview of wound healing; variation in skin pigmentation, healing, and scarring; compares and contrasts beliefs, traditional healing practices, non-Western modalities for wound healing; stigmas and values associated with different types of wounds; suggests implications for nursing practice using a culturally sensitive approach
A culturally congruent diet for Hispanic patients with diabetes	1) Presents national statistics for incidence, complications, and mortality associated with diabetes, contrasting "Hispanic" category with patients who identify as "white, non-Hispanic" 2) Presents Hispanics as one cultural group 3) No discussion of cultural meanings and beliefs associated with different types of food 4) Only presents Mexican foods (e.g., tamales, enchiladas, tacos) as appropriate substitutions on food pyramid 5) No discussion of culturally preferred teaching–learning styles	1) Statistics presented 2) Limitations associated with broad categorization of all Hispanics as a homogenous group discussed 3) Presents table contrasting several different subgroups within Hispanic category, listing common foods, uses, methods of preparation, nutritional value, meaning associated with food 4) Discusses "hot and cold" theory common to most Hispanic groups 5) Case study illustrates cultural pain and distress experienced by a Puerto Rican patient with diabetes who is given a bilingual patient booklet entitled "Diabetic Diets for Mexican Americans" and a second booklet discussing steps to becoming an American citizen

innovations, and re-evaluate within a specified time period. Collaboration with other association members and outside experts will be essential to the overall goals and process. As a second example, an association's program development committee may decide that the annual program topics last year presented cultural competence as an "add-on" or "disconnected attachment." Thereafter, the chosen action will be to connect with a common theme and closing address during the next annual program and re-evaluate.

Certain factors will enhance the ability to conduct an intensive critique. These include psychological factors, practical factors, and expertise factors. Ideally, all conditions should be favorable for a critique to be most successful and valid. Psychological factors include intrinsic motivation, extrinsic motivation, commitment, willingness to make changes, open-mindedness, satisfaction, minimal stress, positive group dynamics, and perceived benefits. Practical factors include time, location and setting, workload, financial resources, board and membership support, bylaws, secretarial support, technical resources, facilities, and energy. Expertise factors include the level of expertise (educational preparation and actual task experience) in evaluation, professional associations, group process, concept mapping, cultural competence development, teaching and learning cultural competence, teaching–learning process, adult learners, culturally diverse members, and learner characteristics.

BARRIERS

Unfortunately, there is a tragic decline in the number of professional association members who have time to serve as volunteers (Shinn, 1998; Skaggs & DeVries, 1998). Furthermore, the number of members with the necessary expertise to conduct a thorough evaluation, propose changes, initiate actions, and implement innovations is sparse. Association leaders will need to recruit, guide, and mentor others in this evaluative process. Undoubtedly, strong, effective leadership is vital to the success of any professional association and its endeavors to facilitate cultural competence development. A major task for professional association leaders is to mentor others as leaders, especially reaching out to nurses who have been traditionally underrepresented in nursing (Bolton et al., 2004; Georges, 2004; Keltner, Kelley, & Smith, 2004; Thompson, 2004; Villarruel & Peragallo, 2004). Appraisal of the association's membership profile in relation to the general population of nurses, neighboring communities, elected leaders within the professional association, and criteria for membership will provide helpful information to guide the association's membership recruitment, retention, and mentoring initiatives. For example, a local chapter of an association whose main mission centers on cultural competence, located in a culturally diverse urban community, should have culturally diverse members representative of the population of nurses and should have culturally diverse qualified elected leaders. (Although recruitment and retention of professional association members is an important issue, it is beyond the scope of this book. Readers are referred to other sources in the literature.)

Another barrier is the devaluing of professional association participation in contrast to other activities. For example, when making tenure and promotion decisions, multidisciplinary committees at universities value a journal publication over service to an association. This is consistent with an individualistic worldview that places the emphasis on individual achievement and accomplishments over group achievements and successes. Although nursing faculty members are expected to belong to professional associations, funding to support memberships, conference fees, and travel is severely limited or virtually nonexistent, especially in public institutions. Similarly, a nurse who agrees to work 4 hours of overtime will receive more positive tacit, indirect, and direct feedback and support from supervisors and colleagues than a nurse who declines to work overtime to attend a professional meeting for 4 hours. Again, the short-term perspective is myopic; it does not examine the long-term benefits that would result from supportive professional development activities such as increased satisfaction and nurse retention. Professional associations today face different challenges than academia and HCIs in finding effective ways of promoting cultural competence development. The level of involvement is confounded by the shortage of nurses and nursing faculty. For example, nursing associations are competing with nurse dissatisfaction in the workplace, fatigue, stress, and time. Nursing associations are also competing with heavy faculty workloads exacerbated by increased nursing student enrollment; lack of sufficient, qualified faculty; and decreased university funds.

Other serious obstacles include the increased proliferation of professional associations, limited numbers of members and resources, duplication of efforts, competition for membership, and high-energy demands in a rapidly changing multicultural society (Shinn, 1998; Skaggs & DeVries, 1998). The question arises as to whether the proliferation of associations has fragmented professional unity and depleted the dynamic energy required to maintain routine activities and invigorate new ideas, explore new directions, stimulate positive change, create new vision, and spark needed innovations within the association and the profession. Furthermore, mandatory membership in a professional association through workplace unions may unintentionally shift focus onto salary, benefits, and workplace conditions rather than on strategies for advancing the science and scholarship of nursing. The challenge is to invigorate, motivate, and involve nurses who initially joined an association because of a unionized workplace to appreciate, value, support, and contribute efforts to advance the nursing profession and cultural competence development.

ACTIONS AND INNOVATIONS

Pacquaio (2004) urged collaboration between associations and agencies in order to capitalize and pool together strengths and expertise, resources to achieve more positive outcomes (success), and avoid duplication of efforts. The idea of joint memberships in professional associations is one option to maximize an association's economic and human resource potential (Shinn, 1998). Often, professional associations have similar missions and attract similar potential members. For example, national ethnic nursing organizations, the Transcultural Nursing Society (international), local chapters of the previous associations, and other similar professional associations share an interest in cultural issues and health care. It takes constant energy to recruit and keep members in any one association and to prevent the recycling of the same members as elected officers and/or task force committee members.

Similarly, local chapters of Sigma Theta Tau, broad professional associations, specialty associations, alumni associations, colleges, and HCIs may also plan events focused on cultural competence development, thus creating further challenges. More cosponsorship of professional events, meetings, and conferences through the ongoing collaborative network development, as well as less (unintentional) competition between activities, will have a more positive effect on participation, energy, fees, attendance, quality, and willingness to volunteer. How successful will any conference be if multiple conferences that generally draw a wide audience of nurses are held in the same city within a few months of each other and/or feature overlapping topics, speakers, and/or agendas? (In such a case, justification to attend more than one conference will be challenging.) Sites of conferences and traveling expenses, time, energy, work release, and distance are important considerations. Examining the existence of supplementary resources available to associations locally, nationally, and internationally is a necessary first step in widely disseminating high-quality educational programs to enhance cultural competence development. The severe nursing shortage further underscores the need to pool resources and share responsibilities within and between associations.

Cultural competence workshops for individuals who realize that cultural competence development is an ongoing, lifelong commitment and who routinely participate in educational pursuits and/or are actively engaged in activities aimed at advancing cultural competence in self and in others serves a valuable purpose. However, these workshops do not reach individuals who are unaware, inefficacious, supremely efficacious, and/or uninterested in cultural competence development. Another challenge is for individuals who are active within associations that prioritize cultural issues to leave their "comfort zone" and venture into new associations less zealous in cultural competence development. Sharing cultural perspectives at meetings, presenting a PowerPoint slideshow or poster that is culturally relevant to the audience, joining committees, and suggesting cosponsorships are some innovations that can be done individually or in groups.

Committees, networking, and mentoring within and between professional associations have a great potential to enhance cultural competence and confidence. As mentioned in chapters 5 and 6, comprehensive understanding, skill, and desire are essential, but not enough to effectively make a positive difference in cultural competence development. The author believes that resilient transcultural self-efficacy (TSE) (confidence) is the integral component necessary in the process of cultural competence development (of self and in others). TSE is the mediating factor that enhances persistence in cultural competence development, despite obstacles, hardships, or stressors. Resilient TSE perceptions embrace lifelong learning in the quest to become "more" culturally competent and in the quest to assist others (learners) in becoming more culturally competent. Professional associations have the potential to develop and nurture resilient TSE perceptions in their members through appropriate educational programs, role modeling, encouragement, and mentoring.

KEY POINT SUMMARY

- Professional associations possess a potentially powerful and extensive ability to network diverse and talented groups of professionals beyond a single health care institution (HCI) or academic setting; therefore, professional associations can exert tremendous influence on promoting, disseminating, and advancing cultural competence development.
- Collectively and individually, professional associations, leaders, and members are challenged to take definitive actions that prioritize and enhance cultural competence development.
- Threads of culture and cultural competency should be equally and substantially evident throughout the association's structure, activities, and resources.

- A systematic evaluation of the association's philosophy and mission, bylaws, membership, newsletter and publications, library, web site, meetings, workshops, conferences, special events, committees, learning strategies, networking, and mentoring helps identify association strengths, weaknesses, inconsistencies, and gaps related to cultural competency development.
- Barriers to maximally enhancing cultural competence development through professional associations include the increased proliferation of professional associations, limited numbers of members and resources, devaluing of professional association activities, duplication of efforts, competition for membership, and high-energy demands in a rapidly changing multicultural society.
- Committees, networking, and mentoring within and between professional associations have a great potential to enhance cultural competence and confidence.
- Professional associations have the potential to develop and nurture resilient TSE perceptions in their members through appropriate educational programs, role modeling, encouragement, and mentoring.

Box 7.1   Educator-in-Action Vignette

Several nurses belonging to the same Nursing Alumni Association engage in an e-mail discussion about upcoming professional conferences. Some excerpts are included:

April: "Next week, on April 15, there is an all-day conference on Meeting Health Care Needs of Diverse Communities at Community Hospital in Urban City, sponsored by the Local Nurses Association. The keynote speaker is Dr. Popular. Are you interested in attending? The conference fee is $60 including lunch and 5 CEs."

Mae: "If I knew ahead of time, I would have requested the day off. Unfortunately, we only get 2 conference days a year. I am on a committee at my Ethnic Nurses' Association. We are planning a cultural conference for May 7. It will be held at the Lodge two streets from Community Hospital. Dr. Popular is also the keynote speaker."

June: "That's interesting. Why didn't I know this before? The rest of the faculty in conjunction with our school's Sigma Theta Tau chapter is sponsoring Cultural Awareness Day on June 15. It will be an all-day symposium in which area nurses involved in projects related to cultural issues will be invited to conduct an oral or poster presentation. We have not decided on a keynote speaker yet; however, Dr. Popular is on the list of potential contacts. I am on the planning committee and also have responsibilities as Chapter Vice President. There are so few volunteers that the planning tasks are overwhelming."

Julie: "Any of those conferences and events sound interesting and I'd like to go. Did you know that the National Association conference theme is focused on culture and health? It is going to be held in Urban City in July, so I can't afford to fly out twice to the same place in such a short time. The budgetary constraints at Public University make it impossible to request funds unless a faculty member is presenting orally at a larger conference. Fortunately, my abstract was accepted. I would have liked to share my study results at any of your association conferences."

Augustino: "Well, I am now hesitant to mention that the regional research alliance has also selected the theme of culture and health. We sent out a call for abstracts in March, but only received 4 by the deadline. The conference is scheduled for August 1–2 in Suburban Town, only 20 minutes outside of Urban City. I am chairperson of the conference planning committee and can't persuade members to join the other three people on the committee. We already put a nonrefundable deposit on the State University's auditorium."

April: "As secretary of State University's Nursing Alumni Association, I am aware that the annual September alumni and student event at State University has invited Dr. Popular to speak about culture and health. It hasn't been officially announced yet. I don't even know if I can attend the event because my clinical specialty nurses' association is having their annual program on the same day in the West Section of Urban City. There should be more discussion about culture and cultural competence within that association."

Conference Results

Each association's conference event is minimally attended. Interested nurses are forced to choose which conference to attend. Active association members on planning committees are exhausted from conference tasks. The thought of planning a future event is overwhelming. Although the majority of the association conferences "break even" between expenses and income generated, two of the associations lose money and only one makes a small profit. The poor attendance discourages potential new members from joining associations.

Future Actions and Innovations

In the future, it will be important to address mutual collaboration, coordination, and cosponsorship of conference events, themes, speakers, and topics to avoid duplication, discourage competition for membership and attendance, promote common professional goals, pool human and financial resources, share responsibilities, and enhance the achievement of conference outcomes.

CHAPTER 8

New Priorities: Challenges and Future Directions

Currently, the process of cultural growth and change (cultural evolution) is strongly influenced by rapid growth in worldwide migration and changes in demographic patterns, marking a new and challenging era for health professionals. More than ever before, health professionals will be expected to provide culturally congruent care to many diverse "culturally different" patients and families. This new era demands a focused, committed, and transformational change that prioritizes cultural competence development through innovative actions guided by systematic inquiry, empirical findings, and conceptual models. This new era necessitates optimism, resilient confidence, and a visionary plan with a prioritized focus.

A first priority is to comprehensively understand the process of becoming cultural competent, recognizing that cultural competence is a multidimensional lifelong learning process rather than a final product. Limited research focused on understanding this "learning" uncovers the need to more fully understand the complex process before jumping ahead and implementing randomized and disconnected teaching interventions. Learning is more than an accumulation of cognitive, practical, and affective skills; learning, persistence for learning, motivation, and skill performance are strongly influenced by psychological factors. Gaining insight into the learner's perceptions will be an essential component to identifying learner's strengths, weaknesses, gaps, and needs.

In this book, the CCC model was proposed as an organizing framework for examining and understanding the multidimensional factors involved in the process of learning cultural competence. TSE (transcultural self-efficacy, meaning the perceived confidence for learning and performing transcultural skills among culturally different patients) is a major influencing factor. The model emphasizes that the cognitive, practical, and affective dimensions of TSE and transcultural skill development can change over time as a result of formalized educational and other learning experiences. In addition, the Transcultural Self-Efficacy Tool (TSET) was proposed as a valid and reliable tool for measuring and evaluating changes in TSE perceptions within the cognitive, practical, and affective domains. The proposed model offers a new theoretical perspective on the process of cultural competence; however, the model is tentative and will require modification with new empirical data. Through the use of the TSET, researchers can further appraise the underlying assumptions and relationships proposed in the model.

A second priority is to creatively design, evaluate, and modify empirically supported educational activities that effectively weave together the main threads of professional life (academia, health care institutions (HCIs), and professional associations) into a resilient fabric that can effectively meet changing climates and unforeseen challenges of the future. Part II of this book suggests strategies for inquiry, action, and innovation within each aspect of professional life; however, educational research remains grossly inadequate in evaluating learner needs and outcomes. The TSET was proposed as a tool for assisting educators in identifying inefficacious learners (at risk for avoiding transcultural skills), identifying supremely efficacious learners (at risk for inadequate preparation for the performance of transcultural skills), and developing diagnostic-prescriptive teaching interventions; ongoing research with the TSET will expand psychometric knowledge and practical application.

This chapter suggests some empirical directions for further systematic inquiry, based on the major areas highlighted in this book. The suggestions are not meant to be exhaustive but are offered with the intent to stimulate new ideas and invite health professionals to explore new paths in the winding journey toward developing cultural competence in self and in others.

FUTURE DIRECTIONS

Theoretical Framework

Studies using constructs, assumptions, and relationships from the CCC model should be conducted across a wide range of settings and health disciplines. Several underlying assumptions about the model have already been supported empirically (Jeffreys, 2000) and have been presented in chapter 3 using the TSET. Quantitative and qualitative studies should be carried out using different groups of students and health professionals to compare similarities and differences based on gender, age, professional experience, ethnicity, race, religion, geographic region, and other demographic variables.

Qualitative Studies

Qualitative studies will add to nursing knowledge by exploring such topics as the following:

- "Lived experience" of learners' changing transcultural perceptions
- Perceived influence of select educational experiences on transcultural skills in the cognitive, practical, and affective dimensions
- Perceived influence of changes in confidence levels and the impact on culturally congruent care, learning, and/or professional satisfaction
- "Lived experience" of promoting, facilitating, and nurturing transcultural learning and self-efficacy in academia, HCIs, or professional associations

Quantitative Studies

Future longitudinal, cross-sectional, or quasi-experimental studies (using the TSET) may help evaluate the effectiveness of select, sequential, integrated, or combined teaching interventions on outcome performances such as culture care competencies, knowledge, skills, patient satisfaction, positive patient outcomes, and confidence. The TSET has been used to

- Identify transcultural skills perceived as more difficult or stressful by learners
- Identify at-risk learners (inefficacious or supremely efficacious/overconfident)
- Develop a composite of learner needs, values, attitudes, and skills concerning transcultural nursing
- Evaluate the effectiveness of teaching interventions
- Assess changes in self-efficacy perceptions over time

The replication of quantitative studies using the TSET will add depth to the beginning knowledge base. Evidence-based educational innovations and ongoing research guided by empirically and conceptually supported literature can effectively guide the transformation necessary to prepare culturally competent health professionals. Researchers should carefully consider which quantitative design and which quantitative measures are most suited for their study purpose and population, especially because funding agencies frequently stipulate the evaluation of outcomes using valid and reliable quantitative measures.

Psychometric Studies

The TSET demonstrated adequate reliability and validity consistently across several studies. Findings supported that the TSET assesses the multidimensional nature of TSE, yet also differentiates between cognitive, practical, and affective learning dimensions. Ongoing psychometric tests of reliability and validity should be incorporated into every study using the TSET because reliability and validity is not an inherent property of the instrument, but only an estimate that may vary among different samples.

Similarly, various scoring and grouping methods proposed in this book (see chapter 3 and appendices E and F) require ongoing testing with various sample populations. Although the TSET was originally designed for undergraduate nursing students and psychometric properties have been explored with several samples of undergraduate nursing students, the instrument has been requested for use and/or adaptation for use with nurses, graduate nursing students, physicians, and other health professionals in various countries. Comparison of psychometric properties across various samples and settings will lend new insight into the possible uses and/or limitations surrounding the instrument. Furthermore, detailed evaluation of adapted and/or translated versions of the instrument will need to be conducted.

Replication

Multiple replications of studies are necessary to assess the reliability of a given construct (Braxton, 2000). Replication with similar and different study samples and settings will add depth to the growing body of knowledge concerning cultural competence and confidence. Developing a program of research that builds on previous findings will enhance understanding about the complex process of cultural competence. Reaching out to other researchers interested in similar studies will permit wider replication among more diverse samples, further expanding knowledge beyond geographic boundaries and settings.

Collaboration and Partnerships

Collaboration between researchers prior to study design and during all phases of the research process will help decrease threats to internal and external validity, as well as promote new ideas and collaborative projects. Developing partnerships between researchers in academia, HCIs, and professional associations will provide the opportunity to connect the wide spectrum of professional activities and roles with a common goal of developing cultural competence and providing culturally congruent care for all culturally diverse patients. In addition, connections within and between disciplines in the United States and beyond will provide another mechanism for reaching out and achieving a broader synthesis for advocating cultural competence beyond the borders often imposed by discipline separation.

CONCLUSION

Societal needs, ethical guidelines, legal issues, and professional goals declare the need to view cultural competence development as a real priority. Such a view necessitates a conscious, committed, and transformational change in current professional practice, education, and research. Individually, every health professional is empowered to positively contribute to this transformational change through an active role in ongoing professional self-development. As active partners, health professionals can continually seek to understand the process of developing cultural competence in self and in others, mentor colleagues, integrate research findings into education and practice, question the status quo, uncover new directions for cultural competence research, implement new innovations, and be open to new ideas. Within purposeful professional partnerships, health professionals will not be alone in the endeavor to promote cultural competence; they will exercise resilience and persist despite challenges and obstacles. Such resilient energy will be maximized through an ongoing open, caring environment that embraces diversity within and between health professions, as well as appreciates diversity within and between patients, families, and communities.

Shaping such an environment amidst managed care, the nursing shortage, faculty shortages, financial constraints, and intergroup and intragroup conflicts presents numerous challenges; however, positive change is possible. Through diligence and coordinated group efforts, the goals of culturally congruent care and multicultural workplace harmony may be achieved. The first step is to step over challenges and open the door to change (see Figure 8.1). Whatever inquiries, actions, and innovations are done (or not done) today will influence the future. Let us join together to make a positive difference through ongoing inquiry, action, and innovation.

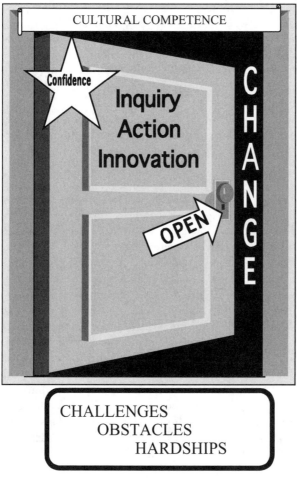

Figure 8.1 Stepping over challenges—opening the door to change.

KEY POINT SUMMARY

- The new era in health care demands a focused, committed, and transformational change that prioritizes cultural competence development.
- A first priority is to comprehensively understand the prcess of becoming culturally competent, recognizing that cultural competence is a multidimensional lifelong learning process rather than a final product.

- A second priority is to creatively design, evaluate, and modify empirically supported teaching–learning strategies that effectively weave together the main threads of professional life (academia, health care institutions, and professional associations) into a resilient fabric that can effectively meet changing climates and unforeseen challenges of the future.
- The CCC model can guide future directions for inquiry, action, and innovation.
- Based on the major areas highlighted in this book, directions for further research include
  - Theoretical framework
  - Qualitative studies
  - Quantitative studies
  - Psychometric studies
  - Replication
  - Collaboration and partnerships

Transcultural Self-Efficacy Tool (TSET)*

*Copyrighted questionnaire. For permission to use TSET, see Appendix I

Throughout your nursing education and nursing career, you will be caring for clients of many different cultural backgrounds. These clients will represent various racial, ethnic, gender, socioeconomic, and religious groups.

Cultural difference exists in health care needs, caring, and curing practices. Knowing and understanding cultural factors related to client care helps establish a theoretical foundation for providing cultural-specific nursing care.

PART I

Among clients of *different* culture backgrounds, how knowledgeable are *YOU* about the ways cultural factors may influence nursing care? Please use the following scale and mark your response accordingly.

You know and understand the ways *cultural factors* may influence *nursing care* in the following areas:

	Not Confident 1	2	3	4	5	6	7	8	9	Totally Confident 10
1) health history and interview	1	2	3	4	5	6	7	8	9	10
2) physical examination	1	2	3	4	5	6	7	8	9	10
3) informed consent	1	2	3	4	5	6	7	8	9	10
4) health promotion	1	2	3	4	5	6	7	8	9	10
5) illness prevention	1	2	3	4	5	6	7	8	9	10
6) health maintenance	1	2	3	4	5	6	7	8	9	10
7) health restoration	1	2	3	4	5	6	7	8	9	10
8) safety	1	2	3	4	5	6	7	8	9	10
9) exercise and activity	1	2	3	4	5	6	7	8	9	10

	1	2	3	4	5	6	7	8	9	10
10) pain relief and comfort	①	②	③	④	⑤	⑥	⑦	⑧	⑨	⑩
11) diet and nutrition	①	②	③	④	⑤	⑥	⑦	⑧	⑨	⑩
12) patient teaching	①	②	③	④	⑤	⑥	⑦	⑧	⑨	⑩
13) hygiene	①	②	③	④	⑤	⑥	⑦	⑧	⑨	⑩
14) anxiety and stress reduction	①	②	③	④	⑤	⑥	⑦	⑧	⑨	⑩
15) diagnostic tests	①	②	③	④	⑤	⑥	⑦	⑧	⑨	⑩
16) blood tests	①	②	③	④	⑤	⑥	⑦	⑧	⑨	⑩
17) pregnancy	①	②	③	④	⑤	⑥	⑦	⑧	⑨	⑩
18) birth	①	②	③	④	⑤	⑥	⑦	⑧	⑨	⑩
19) growth and development	①	②	③	④	⑤	⑥	⑦	⑧	⑨	⑩
20) aging	①	②	③	④	⑤	⑥	⑦	⑧	⑨	⑩
21) dying and death	①	②	③	④	⑤	⑥	⑦	⑧	⑨	⑩
22) grieving and loss	①	②	③	④	⑤	⑥	⑦	⑧	⑨	⑩
23) life support and resuscitation	①	②	③	④	⑤	⑥	⑦	⑧	⑨	⑩
24) sexuality	①	②	③	④	⑤	⑥	⑦	⑧	⑨	⑩
25) rest and sleep	①	②	③	④	⑤	⑥	⑦	⑧	⑨	⑩

PART II

The most effective way to identify specific cultural factors that influence client behavior is to conduct a cultural assessment of each client. This is best done by interview.

Right NOW, how confident are *YOU* about *interviewing clients of different cultural backgrounds* to learn about their values and beliefs?

Rate your degree of confidence or certainty for each of the following *interview topics*. Please use the following scale and mark your response accordingly.

Interview clients of different cultural backgrounds about:

	Not Confident									Totally Confident
	①	②	③	④	⑤	⑥	⑦	⑧	⑨	⑩
26) language preference	①	②	③	④	⑤	⑥	⑦	⑧	⑨	⑩
27) level of English comprehension	①	②	③	④	⑤	⑥	⑦	⑧	⑨	⑩
28) meaning of verbal communication patterns	①	②	③	④	⑤	⑥	⑦	⑧	⑨	⑩
29) meaning of nonverbal behaviors	①	②	③	④	⑤	⑥	⑦	⑧	⑨	⑩
30) meanings of space and touch	①	②	③	④	⑤	⑥	⑦	⑧	⑨	⑩
31) time perception and orientation	①	②	③	④	⑤	⑥	⑦	⑧	⑨	⑩
32) racial background and identity	①	②	③	④	⑤	⑥	⑦	⑧	⑨	⑩
33) ethnic background and identity	①	②	③	④	⑤	⑥	⑦	⑧	⑨	⑩
34) socioeconomic background	①	②	③	④	⑤	⑥	⑦	⑧	⑨	⑩
35) religious background and identity	①	②	③	④	⑤	⑥	⑦	⑧	⑨	⑩
36) educational background and interests	①	②	③	④	⑤	⑥	⑦	⑧	⑨	⑩

	1	2	3	4	5	6	7	8	9	10
37) religious practices and beliefs	①	②	③	④	⑤	⑥	⑦	⑧	⑨	⑩
38) acculturation	①	②	③	④	⑤	⑥	⑦	⑧	⑨	⑩
39) worldview (philosophy of life)	①	②	③	④	⑤	⑥	⑦	⑧	⑨	⑩
40) attitudes about health care technology	①	②	③	④	⑤	⑥	⑦	⑧	⑨	⑩
41) ethnic food preferences	①	②	③	④	⑤	⑥	⑦	⑧	⑨	⑩
42) role of elders	①	②	③	④	⑤	⑥	⑦	⑧	⑨	⑩
43) role of children	①	②	③	④	⑤	⑥	⑦	⑧	⑨	⑩
44) financial concerns	①	②	③	④	⑤	⑥	⑦	⑧	⑨	⑩
45) traditional health and illness beliefs	①	②	③	④	⑤	⑥	⑦	⑧	⑨	⑩
46) folk medicine tradition and use	①	②	③	④	⑤	⑥	⑦	⑧	⑨	⑩
47) gender role and responsibility	①	②	③	④	⑤	⑥	⑦	⑧	⑨	⑩
48) acceptable sick role behaviors	①	②	③	④	⑤	⑥	⑦	⑧	⑨	⑩
49) role of family during illness	①	②	③	④	⑤	⑥	⑦	⑧	⑨	⑩
50) discrimination and bias experiences	①	②	③	④	⑤	⑥	⑦	⑧	⑨	⑩
51) home environment	①	②	③	④	⑤	⑥	⑦	⑧	⑨	⑩
52) kinship ties	①	②	③	④	⑤	⑥	⑦	⑧	⑨	⑩
53) aging	①	②	③	④	⑤	⑥	⑦	⑧	⑨	⑩

PART III

As a nurse who will care for many different people, *knowledge of yourself* is very important.
Please rate *YOUR* degree of confidence or certainty for each of the following items. Use the following scale and mark your response accordingly.

	Not Confident									Totally Confident
	①	②	③	④	⑤	⑥	⑦	⑧	⑨	⑩

A) About yourself, you are *AWARE OF:*

54) *YOUR OWN* cultural heritage and belief systems	①	②	③	④	⑤	⑥	⑦	⑧	⑨	⑩
55) *YOUR OWN* biases and limitations	①	②	③	④	⑤	⑥	⑦	⑧	⑨	⑩
56) differences within *YOUR OWN* cultural group	①	②	③	④	⑤	⑥	⑦	⑧	⑨	⑩

B) *Among clients of different cultural backgrounds,*
  You are *AWARE OF:*

57) insensitive and prejudicial treatment	①	②	③	④	⑤	⑥	⑦	⑧	⑨	⑩
58) differences in perceived role of the nurse	①	②	③	④	⑤	⑥	⑦	⑧	⑨	⑩
59) traditional caring behaviors	①	②	③	④	⑤	⑥	⑦	⑧	⑨	⑩
60) professional caring behaviors	①	②	③	④	⑤	⑥	⑦	⑧	⑨	⑩

168

	1	2	3	4	5	6	7	8	9	10
61) comfort and discomfort felt when entering a culturally different world	①	②	③	④	⑤	⑥	⑦	⑧	⑨	⑩
62) interaction between nursing, folk, and professional systems	①	②	③	④	⑤	⑥	⑦	⑧	⑨	⑩
You *ACCEPT*:										
63) differences between cultural groups	①	②	③	④	⑤	⑥	⑦	⑧	⑨	⑩
64) similarities between cultural groups	①	②	③	④	⑤	⑥	⑦	⑧	⑨	⑩
65) client's refusal for treatment based on beliefs	①	②	③	④	⑤	⑥	⑦	⑧	⑨	⑩
You *APPRECIATE*:										
66) interaction with people of different cultures	①	②	③	④	⑤	⑥	⑦	⑧	⑨	⑩
67) cultural sensitivity and awareness	①	②	③	④	⑤	⑥	⑦	⑧	⑨	⑩
68) cultural-specific nursing care	①	②	③	④	⑤	⑥	⑦	⑧	⑨	⑩
69) role of family in providing health care	①	②	③	④	⑤	⑥	⑦	⑧	⑨	⑩
70) client's worldview (philosophy of life)	①	②	③	④	⑤	⑥	⑦	⑧	⑨	⑩
You *RECOGNIZE*:										
71) inadequacies in the U.S. health care system	①	②	③	④	⑤	⑥	⑦	⑧	⑨	⑩
72) importance of home remedies and folk medicine	①	②	③	④	⑤	⑥	⑦	⑧	⑨	⑩
73) impact of roles on health care practices	①	②	③	④	⑤	⑥	⑦	⑧	⑨	⑩

(*continued*)

	Not Confident									Totally Confident
	①	②	③	④	⑤	⑥	⑦	⑧	⑨	⑩

Among clients of different cultural backgrounds,

You **RECOGNIZE:**

	①	②	③	④	⑤	⑥	⑦	⑧	⑨	⑩
74) impact of values on health care practices	①	②	③	④	⑤	⑥	⑦	⑧	⑨	⑩
75) impact of socioeconomic factors on health care practices	①	②	③	④	⑤	⑥	⑦	⑧	⑨	⑩
76) impact of political factors on health care practices	①	②	③	④	⑤	⑥	⑦	⑧	⑨	⑩
77) need for cultural care preservation/ maintenance	①	②	③	④	⑤	⑥	⑦	⑧	⑨	⑩
78) need for cultural care accommodation/ negotiation	①	②	③	④	⑤	⑥	⑦	⑧	⑨	⑩
79) need for cultural care repatterning/ restructuring	①	②	③	④	⑤	⑥	⑦	⑧	⑨	⑩
80) need to prevent ethnocentric views	①	②	③	④	⑤	⑥	⑦	⑧	⑨	⑩
81) need to prevent cultural imposition	①	②	③	④	⑤	⑥	⑦	⑧	⑨	⑩

You **ADVOCATE:**

	①	②	③	④	⑤	⑥	⑦	⑧	⑨	⑩
82) client's decisions based on cultural beliefs	①	②	③	④	⑤	⑥	⑦	⑧	⑨	⑩
83) cultural-specific care	①	②	③	④	⑤	⑥	⑦	⑧	⑨	⑩

APPENDIX B

Cognitive Subscale: Item Overview

Cognitive (Know and Understand Ways Cultural Factors May Influence Nursing Care)

Professional Nursing Care

Health history and interview
Physical exam*
Informed consent*
Health promotion*
Illness prevention*
Health maintenance*
Health restoration*
Safety*
Exercise and activity*
Pain relief and comfort*
Rest and sleep
Diet and nutrition
Patient teaching
Hygiene
Anxiety and stress reduction
Diagnostic tests
Blood tests

Life Cycle Transitional Phenomena

Pregnancy*
Birth*
Sexuality*
Growth and development*
Aging*
Dying and death*
Grieving and loss*
Life support and resuscitation*

*Items loaded on specified factors exclusively in factor analysis study (Jeffreys & Smodlaka, 1998).

Practical Subscale: Item Overview

Practical* (Interview Clients of Different Cultural Backgrounds)

Communication

Language preference
Level of English comprehension
Meaning of verbal communication patterns
Meaning of nonverbal communication patterns
Meanings of space and touch
Time perception and orientation

Cultural Background and Identity

Ethnic background and identity
Religious background and identity
Socioeconomic background
Religious background and identity
Religious practices and beliefs
Educational background and interests
Acculturation
Worldview (philosophy of life)
Attitudes about health care technology

Kinship and Social Factors

Role of elders
Role of children
Role of family during illness
Acceptable sick role behaviors
Gender role and responsibilities
Traditional health and illness beliefs
Folk medicine tradition and use
Home environment
Kinship ties
Aging
Discrimination and bias experiences
Ethnic food preferences
Financial concerns

*All items loaded on specified factors exclusively in factor analysis study (Jeffreys & Smodlaka, 1998).

Affective Subscale: Item Overview

Affective   (Values, Attitudes, and Beliefs)

Self-Awareness

Own cultural heritage and belief systems*
Own biases and limitations*
Differences within own cultural group*

Among clients of different cultural backgrounds

Awareness

Insensitive and prejudicial treatment*
Differences in perceived role of the nurse*
Traditional caring behaviors*
Professional caring behaviors*
Comfort and discomfort felt when entering a culturally different world*
Interaction between nursing, folk, and professional systems*

Acceptance

Difference between cultural groups
Similarities between cultural groups
Client's refusal of treatment based on beliefs

Appreciation

Interaction with people of different cultures*
Cultural sensitivity and awareness*
Cultural-specific nursing care*
Role of family in providing health care*
Client's worldview (philosophy of life)*

Recognition

Inadequacies in the U.S. health care system*
Importance of home remedies and folk medicine*

(*continued*)

Impact of roles on health care practices*
Impact of values on health care practices*
Impact of socioeconomic factors on health care practices*
Impact of political factors on health care practices*
Need for cultural care preservation/maintenance*
Need for cultural care accommodation/negotiation*
Need for cultural care repatterning/restructuring*
Need to prevent ethnocentric views*
Need to prevent cultural imposition*

Advocacy

Client's decisions based on cultural beliefs
Cultural-specific care

---

*Items loaded on specified factors exclusively in factor analysis study (Jeffreys & Smodlaka, 1998).

Scoring Information

TRANSCULTURAL SELF-EFFICACY TOOL

Scoring Suggestions

Consistent with many other self-efficacy instruments, scoring of the Transcultural Self-Efficacy Tool (TSET) includes subscale calculations of self-efficacy strength (SEST) and self-efficacy level (SEL).

SEST refers to the average strength of self-efficacy perceptions within a particular dimension (subscale) of the construct. On the TSET, SEST scores are calculated by totaling subscale item responses and dividing by the number of subscale items, resulting in the mean score. SEST scores are used most often in self-efficacy studies.

SEL refers to the number of items perceived at a specified minimum level of confidence. For example, SEL has been used to identify individuals with "low efficacy" and then track SEL changes following treatment interventions. The study purpose and sample may guide the selected definition of the minimum confidence level. (See chapter 3.)

Grouping samples into low, medium, and high efficacy groups based on SEST, SEL, and/or some other criterion permits further comparative analyses and the identification of at-risk individuals (inefficacious and supremely efficacious). Several different methods may be used for group categorization and comparison, such as plus or minus one standard deviation of sample's subscale mean or defining score ranges for low, medium, and high groups. (See chapter 3.)

TSET Application

In summary, calculation of SEST scores for each TSET subscale is routinely recommended whenever the TSET is used. TSET SEL scores are an additional, supplemental approach for analyzing data. Different methods can be employed to group individuals into low, medium, and high efficacy groups for the purpose of identifying at-risk individuals and tracking changes. The study purpose and sample may guide method selection for group categorization.

Contact author for further scoring information:
Dr. Marianne R. Jeffreys
The City University of New York
College of Staten Island
Nursing Department

Sample Methods for Categorizing Low, High, and Medium Groups

		Cognitive Subscale	Practical Subscale	Affective Subscale
Method 1				
Low	Select 1 or 2 responses on 80% or + items	5 or more items	6 or more items	5 or more items
High	Select 9 or 10 responses on 80% or + items	20 or more items	24 or more items	23 or more items
Medium	Select 3 through 8 responses on 80% items or does not fall into low or high group*	6 to 19 items or *	7 to 23 items or *	6 to 22 items or *
Method 2				
Low	SEL below subscale maximum possible SEL	SEL below 25	SEL below 30	SEL below 28
High	Select 9 or 10 on all subscale items	9 or 10 on 25 items	9 or 10 on 30 items	9 or 10 on 28 items
Medium	Respondents who do not fall into low or high group*	*	*	*
Method 3				
Low	Sum subscale responses < 20% maximum total	Sum ≤ 50	Sum ≤ 60	Sum ≤ 56
High	Sum subscale responses indicate ≥ 9 or 10 response selection exclusively for each subscale item	Sum ≥ 22.5	Sum ≥ 270	Sum ≥ 252
Medium	Respondents who do not fall into low or high group*	*	*	*
Method 4				
Low	SEL below subscale maximum possible SEL	SEL below 25	SEL below 30	SEL below 28
High	Sum subscale responses indicate ≥ 9 or 10 response selection exclusively for each subscale item	Sum ≥ 225	Sum ≥ 270	Sum ≥ 252
Medium	Respondents who do not fall into low or high group*	*	*	*
Method 5				
Low	Below −1.0 standard deviation (SD) of subscale mean	SEST < −1.0 SD	SEST < −1.0 SD	SEST < −1.0 SD
High	Above +1.0 SD of subscale mean	SEST > +1.0 SD	SEST > +1.0 SD	SEST > +1.0 SD
Medium	Within ±1.0 SD of subscale mean	SEST = ±1.0 SD	SEST = ±1.0 SD	SEST = ±1.0 SD
Method 6				
Low	Lowest 33.3% of SEST subscale scores	SEST lowest 33.3%	SEST lowest 33.3%	SEST lowest 33.3%
High	Highest 33.3% of SEST subscale scores	SEST highest 33.3%	SEST highest 33.3%	SEST highest 33.3%
Medium	Middle 33.3% of SEST subscale scores	SEST middle 33.3%	SEST middle 33.3%	SEST middle 33.3%
Method 7				
Low	Lowest 25% of SEST subscale scores	SEST lowest 25%	SEST lowest 25%	SEST lowest 25%
High	Highest 25% of SEST subscale scores	SEST highest 25%	SEST highest 25%	SEST highest 25%
Medium	Middle 50% of SEST subscale scores	SEST middle 50%	SEST middle 50%	SEST middle 50%

*Only Method 1 was tested with undergraduate nursing students and nurses. Other methods are proposed as other options. See chapter 3 for suggestions and details.

Sample Demographic Data Potentially Relevant for Collection With the Transcultural Self-Efficacy Tool: Nursing Students

BACKGROUND INFORMATION

Please mark one choice for each item:

1) Name of Institution:
   - ○ College A   ○ College E
   - ○ College B   ○ College F
   - ○ College C   ○ College G
   - ○ College D   ○ College H

2) Current clinical nursing course enrolled in:
   - ○ First semester
   - ○ Second semester
   - ○ Third semester
   - ○ Fourth semester

3) This clinical nursing course deals with:
   - ○ Medical–surgical (adult health)   ○ Community health
   - ○ Psychiatric (mental health)   ○ Critical care
   - ○ Maternity (pregnancy, childbirth)   ○ Pediatric (child and adolescent)

4) Gender
   - ○ Female   ○ Male

5) Age
   - ○ Under 25   ○ 45–49
   - ○ 25–29   ○ 50–54
   - ○ 30–34   ○ 55–59
   - ○ 35–39   ○ 60 and over
   - ○ 40–44

6) Which of the following categories best describes you?
   (May select more than one choice)
   - ○ Alaskan Native or American Indian   ○ Black
   - ○ Asian or Pacific Islander   ○ White
   - ○ Puerto Rican   ○ Other
   - ○ Other Hispanic

7) Is English your first language?
   - ○ Yes   ○ No

8) Family's total yearly income before taxes:
   - ○ Less than $9,000   ○ $35,000–$44,999
   - ○ $9,000–$14,999   ○ $45,000–$54,999
   - ○ $15,000–$19,999   ○ $55,000–$64,999
   - ○ $20,000–$24,999   ○ $65,000–$74,999
   - ○ $25,000–$34,999   ○ $75,000 and above

9) Previous health care experience:
   - ○ None
   - ○ LPN
   - ○ Other

Sample Demographic Data Potentially Relevant for Collection With the Transcultural Self-Efficacy Tool: Registered Nurses

BACKGROUND INFORMATION

Please mark one choice for each item:

1) Gender
   - ○ Female   ○ Male

2) Age
   - ○ Under 25   ○ 45–49
   - ○ 25–29   ○ 50–54
   - ○ 30–34   ○ 55–59
   - ○ 35–39   ○ 60 and over
   - ○ 40–44

3) Which of the following categories best describes you?
   (May select more than one choice)
   - ○ Alaskan Native or American Indian   ○ Black
   - ○ Asian or Pacific Islander   ○ White
   - ○ Puerto Rican   ○ Other
   - ○ Other Hispanic

4) Is English your first language?
   - ○ Yes   ○ No

5) Health care setting in which you presently work:
   - ○ Hospital (acute care)   ○ School
   - ○ Hospital (chronic care)   ○ Occupational health
   - ○ Clinic   ○ School of nursing
   - ○ Nursing home   ○ Hospice
   - ○ Home care   ○ Other

6) Clinical area in which you presently work:
   - ○ Medical–surgical   ○ Geriatric
   - ○ Oncology   ○ Rehabilitation
   - ○ Psychiatric   ○ Substance abuse
   - ○ Maternal–child   ○ HIV and AIDS
   - ○ Emergency   ○ Other

7) Nursing position that you currently hold:
   - ○ Staff RN   ○ Nurse entrepreneur
   - ○ Assistant head nurse   ○ Research nurse
   - ○ Nurse manager/head nurse   ○ Private duty RN
   - ○ Nurse educator   ○ None (unemployed)
   - ○ Nurse administrator/supervisor ○ Other

8) How many years have you been licensed as a registered nurse?
   - ○ Under 2   ○ 20–24
   - ○ 2–4   ○ 25–29
   - ○ 5–9   ○ 30–34
   - ○ 10–14   ○ 35–39
   - ○ 15–19   ○ 40 or more

9) What type of *initial* nursing program did you complete?
   - ○ Associate's degree (university based)   ○ Master's degree
   - ○ Associate's degree (hospital based)   ○ Other program (foreign)
   - ○ Diploma program (hospital based)   ○ Other program (U.S.)
   - ○ Baccalaureate degree

APPENDIX I

Sample Permission Letter

Requester's Name and Credentials
Mailing Address
E-mail Address
Date

Permissions Editor
Springer Publishing Company
11 West 42nd Street
New York, New York 10036-8002

Dear Publisher:

I am writing to request permission to use the Transcultural Self-Efficacy Tool (TSET) in my research study. The study addresses _____ (briefly describe nature of study, purpose, sample, etc.).

I have mailed a copy of this request letter to the author:

> Dr. Marianne R. Jeffreys
> The City University of New York College of Staten Island
> Nursing Department
> 2800 Victory Boulevard
> Staten Island, New York 10314

I also agree to send Dr. Jeffreys further reliability and validity test results for the TSET at the above address.

Sincerely,

Signature

Name, Credentials

Title

References

Abrums, M. E., & Leppa, C. (2001). Beyond cultural competence: Teaching about race, gender, class, and sexual orientation. *Journal of Nursing Education, 40*(6), 270–275.

Adams, C. E., Murdock, J. E., Valiga, T. M., McGinnis, S., & Wolfertz, J. R. (2002). *Trends in registered nurse education programs: A comparison across three points in time—1994; 1999; 2004.* Retrieved April 2, 2003, from http://www.nln.org/aboutnln/nursetrends.htm.

American Nurses Association (ANA). (1991). *Position statement on cultural diversity in nursing practice.* Retrieved January 30, 2005, from http://nursingworld.org/readroom/position/ethics/etcldv.htm.

American Nurses Association (ANA). (1998). *Position statement on discrimination and racism in health care.* Retrieved January 30, 2005, from http://nursingworld.org/readroom/position/ethics/etdisrac.htm.

American Nurses Association (ANA). (2001). *Code for nurses with interpretive statements.* Washington, DC: Author.

American Nurses Association (ANA). (2003). *Nursing's social policy statement* (2nd ed.). Washington, DC: Author.

American Nurses Association (ANA). (2004). *Nursing: Scope and standards of practice.* Washington, DC: Author.

Andrews, M. (1995). Transcultural nursing: Transforming the curriculum. *Journal of Transcultural Nursing, 6*(2), 4–9.

Andrews, M. M., & Boyle, J. S. (2002). *Transcultural concepts in nursing care* (4th ed.). Philadelphia: Lippincott Williams & Wilkins.

Andrews, M., & Boyle, J. (1999). *Transcultural concepts in nursing* (3rd ed.). Philadelphia: Lippincott.

Andrews, M., Burr, J., & Janetos, D. H. (2004). Searching electronically for information on transcultural nursing and health subjects. *Journal of Transcultural Nursing, 15*(3), 242–247.

Antonio, A. L. (2001). Diversity and the influence of friendship groups in college. *Review of Higher Education, 25*(1), 63–89.

Baker, C. R. (2001). Role strain in male diploma nursing students: A descriptive quantitative study. *Journal of Nursing Education, 40*(8), 378–380.

Baldwin, D. (1999). Community-based experiences and cultural competence. *Journal of Nursing Education, 38*(5), 195–196.

Bandura, A. (1977). Self-efficacy: Toward a unifying theory of behavioral change. *Psychological Review, 84*(2), 191–215.

Bandura, A. (1982). Self-efficacy mechanism in human agency. *American Psychologist, 37*(2), 122–145.

Bandura, A. (1986). *Social foundations of thought and action: A social cognitive theory.* Englewood Cliffs, NJ: Prentice Hall.

Bandura, A. (1989). Regulation of cognitive processes through perceived self-efficacy. *Developmental Psychology, 25*(5), 729–735.

Bandura, A. (1995). On rectifying conceptual ecumenism. In J. E. Maddux (Ed.), *Self-efficacy, adaptation, and adjustment: Theory, research, and application* (pp. 347–375). New York: Plenum.

Bandura, A. (1996a). Reflections on human agency. In J. Georgas, M. Manthouli, E. Besevegis, & A. Kokkevi (Eds.), *Contemporary psychology in Europe: Theory, research, and applications. Proceedings of the IVth European Congress of Psychology* (pp. 194–210). Seattle, WA: Hogrefe & Huber.

Bandura, A. (1996b). Regulation of cognitive processes through perceived self-efficacy. In G-H. Jennings (Ed.), *Passages beyond the gate: A Jungian approach to understanding the nature of American psychology at the dawn of the new millennium* (pp. 96–107). Needham Heights, MA: Simon & Schuster.

Bandura, A. (1997). *Self-efficacy: The exercise of control.* New York: W. H. Freeman.

Bandura, A., & Schunk, D. H. (1981). Cultivating competence, self-efficacy and intrinsic interest through proximal self-motivation. *Journal of Personality and Social Psychology, 41*, 586–598.

Barbee, E. L., & Gibson, S. E. (2001). Our dismal progress: The recruitment of non-whites into nursing. *Journal of Nursing Education, 40*(6), 243–245.

Bernal, H., & Froman, R. (1987). The confidence of community health nurses in caring for ethnically diverse populations. *Image: Journal of Nursing Scholarship, 19*, 201–203.

Berry, J. M., West, R. L., & Dennehey, D. M. (1989). Reliability and validity of memory self-efficacy questionnaire. *Developmental Psychology, 25*, 701–713.

Bessent, H. (1997). *Strategies for recruitment, retention, and graduation of minority nurses in colleges of nursing.* Washington, DC: American Nurses Publishing.

Betts, V. T., & Cherry, B. (2002). Health policy and politics. In B. Cherry & S. R. Jacob (Eds.), *Contemporary nursing: Issues, trends, and management* (2nd ed., pp. 219–235). Philadelphia: Mosby.

Bibb, S. C., Malebranche, M., Crowell, D., Altman, C., Lyon, S., Carlson, A., Miller, S., Miller, T., & Rybarczyk, J. (2003). Professional development needs of registered nurses practicing at a military community hospital. *Journal of Continuing Education in Nursing, 34*(1), 39–45.

Bilinski, H. (2002). The mentored journal. *Nurse Educator, 27*(1), 37–41.

Billings, D. (2004). Teaching learners from varied generations. *Journal of Continuing Education in Nursing, 35*(3), 104–105.

Bloom, B. S., Englehart, M. D., Furst, E. J., Hill, W. H., & Krathwohl, D. R. (1956). *Taxonomy of educational objectives: Handbook I: Cognitive domain.* New York: McKay.

Bolan, C. M. (2003). Incorporating the experiential learning theory into the instructional design of online courses. *Nurse Educator, 28*(1), 10–14.

Bolton, L. B., Giger, J. N., & Georges, C. A. (2004). Structural and racial barriers to health care. In L. Fitzpatrick (Ed.), *Annual review of nursing research* (Vol. 22, pp. 39–58). New York: Springer Publishing.

Bolton, L. B. (2004). Cultural diversity in leadership. *Nursing Administration Quarterly, 28*(3), 163–164.

Boyce, B. A. B., & Winne, M. D. (2000). Developing an evaluation tool for instructional software programs. *Nurse Educator, 25*(3), 145–148.

Braxton, J. M. (2000). Reinvigorating theory & research on the departure puzzle. In J. M. Braxton (Ed.), *Reworking the student departure puzzle* (pp. 257–274). Nashville, TN: Vanderbilt University Press.

Brookfield, S. D. (1986). *Understanding and facilitating adult learning.* San Francisco: Jossey-Bass.

Brown, S. D., Lent, R. W., & Larkin, K. C. (1989). Self-efficacy as a moderator of scholastic aptitude: Academic performance relationships. *Journal of Vocational Behavior, 35*(1), 64–75.

Burr, P. L., Burr, R. M., & Novak, L. F. (1999). Student retention is more complicated than merely keeping the students you have today: Toward a "seamless retention theory." *Journal of College Student Retention, 1*(3), 239–253.

Callister, L. C., Khalaf, I., & Keller, D. (2000). Cross-cultural comparison of the concerns of beginning baccalaureate nursing students. *Nurse Educator, 25*(6), 267–271.

Cameron-Traub, E. (2002). Western ethical, moral, and legal dimensions within the culture care theory. In M. Leininger & M. McFarland (Eds.), *Transcultural nursing: Concepts, theories, research, and practice* (pp. 169–177). New York: McGraw-Hill.

Campinha-Bacote, J. (1998). *The process of cultural competence in the delivery of healthcare services: A culturally competent model of care* (3rd ed.). Cincinnati, OH: Transcultural C.A.R.E. Associates.

Campinha-Bacote, J. (1999). A model and instrument for addressing cultural competence in health care. *Journal of Nursing Education, 38,* 203–207.

Campinha-Bacote, J. (2003). *The process of cultural competence in the delivery of healthcare services: A culturally competent model of care* (4th ed.). Cincinnati, OH: Transcultural C.A.R.E. Associates.

Candela, L., Michael, S. R., & Mitchell, S. (2003). Ethical debates: Enhancing critical thinking in nursing students. *Nurse Educator, 28*(1), 37–39.

Carmines, E., & Zeller, R. A. (1979). *Reliability and validity assessment.* Newbury Park, CA: Sage.

Cavanaugh, D. A., & Huse, A. L. (2004). Surviving the nursing shortage: Developing a nursing orientation program to prepare and retain intensive care unit nurses. *Journal of Continuing Education in Nursing, 35*(6), 251–256.

Cervone, D. (1989). Effects of envisioning future activities on self-efficacy judgments and motivation: An availability heuristic interpretation. *Cognitive Therapy and Research, 13*(3), 247–260.

Cervone, D., & Palmer, B. W. (1990). Anchoring biases and the perseverence of self-efficacy beliefs. *Cognitive Therapy & Research, 14*(4), 401–416.

Cervone, D., & Peake, P. K. (1986). Anchoring, efficacy, and action: The influence of judgmental heuristics on self-efficacy judgments & behavior. *Journal of Personality & Social Psychology, 50*, 492–501.

Chang, M. K. (1995). Bridging the cultural gap. *Urologic Nursing, 15*(14), 123–126.

Chartrand, J. M. (1990). A causal analysis to predict the personal and academic adjustment of nontraditional students. *Journal of Counseling Psychology, 37*(1), 65–73.

Christiaens, G., & Baldwin, J. H. (2002). Use of dyadic role-playing to increase student participation. *Nurse Educator, 27*(6), 251–254.

Christianson, L., Tiene, D., & Luft, P. (2002). Web-based teaching in undergraduate nursing programs. *Journal of Nursing Education, 27*(6), 276–282.

Cohen, J. (1977). *Statistical power analysis for the behavioral sciences* (Rev. ed.). New York: Academic Press.

Collins, J. M. (2002). Reflections on the changing learning needs of nurses: A challenge for nursing continuing educators. *Journal of Continuing Education in Nursing, 33*(2), 74–77.

Comrey, A. L. (1973). *A first course in factor analysis.* New York: Academic Press.

Constantine, M. G., & Watt, S. K. (2002). Cultural congruity, womanist identity attitudes, and life satisfaction among African American college women attending historically black and predominantly white institutions. *Journal of College Student Development, 43*(2), 184–193.

Constantine, M. G., Robinson, J. S., Wilton, L., & Caldwell, L. D. (2002). Collective self-esteem and perceived social support as predictors of cultural congruity among black and Latino college students. *Journal of College Student Development, 43*(3), 307–316.

Courage, M. M., & Godbey, K. L. (1992). Student retention: Policies and services to enhance persistence to graduation. *Nurse Educator, 17*(2), 29–32.

Cowen, K. J., & Tesh, A. S. (2002). Effects of gaming on nursing students' knowledge of pediatric cardiovascular dysfunction. *Journal of Nursing Education, 41*(11), 507–509.

Crow, K. (1993). Multiculturalism and pluralistic thought in nursing education: Native American world view and the nursing academic world view. *Journal of Nursing Education, 32*(5), 198–204.

Cummings, P. H. (1998). Nursing in Barbados: A fourth-year elective practice experience for nursing students and registered nurses. *Journal of Nursing Education, 37*(1), 42–44.

Daniel, G. R. (1992). Beyond black and white: The new multiracial consciousness. In M. P. P. Root (Ed.), *Racially mixed people in America* (pp. 333–341). Newbury Park, CA: Sage.

Davidhizar, R., Dowd, S. B., & Giger, J. N. (1998). Educating the culturally diverse healthcare student. *Nurse Educator, 23*(2), 38–42.

Davidson, P. M., Meleis, A., Daly, J., & Douglas, M. (2003). Globalisation as we enter the 21st century: Reflections and directions for nursing education, science, research and clinical practice. *Contemporary Nurse, 15*(3), 162–174.

Dearman, C. N. (2003). Using clinical scenarios in nursing education. In M. Oermann & K. Heinrich (Eds.), *Annual review of nursing education* (Vol. I, pp. 341–355). New York: Springer Publishing.

Delgado, C., & Mack, B. (2002). A peer-reviewed program for senior proficiencies. *Nurse Educator, 27*(5), 212–213.

Department of Health and Human Services (DHHS). (2000). *Healthy People 2010: Understanding and improving health* (2nd ed.). Washington, DC: U.S. Government Printing Office.

Diekelmann, N. (2002). "She asked this simple question": Reflecting and the scholarship of teaching. *Journal of Nursing Education, 41*(9), 381–382.

Diekelmann, N., & Ironside, P. M. (2002). Developing a science of nursing education: Innovation with research. *Journal of Nursing Education, 41*(9), 379–380.

DiMaria-Ghalili, R. A., Ostrow, L., & Rodney, K. (2005). Webcasting: A new instructional technology in distance graduate nursing education. *Journal of Nursing Education, 44*(1), 11–18.

Dolgan, C. M. (2001). *The effects of cultural competency training on nurses' attitudes*. Unpublished master's thesis, Cleveland State University, Cleveland, OH.

Donnelly, P. J. L. (1992). The impact of culture on psychotherapy: Korean clients' expectations in psychotherapy, *Journal of the New York State Nurses Association, 23*(2), 12–19.

Donnelly, P. J. L. (2005). Mental health beliefs and help seeking behaviors of Korean American parents of adult children with schizophrenia. *Journal of Multicultural Nursing and Health, 11*(2), 23–24.

Douglas, M. (2000). The effect of globalization on health care: A double-edged sword. *Journal of Transcultural Nursing, 11*(2), 85–86.

Drevdahl, D. J., Stackman, R. W., Purdy, J. M., & Louie, B. Y. (2002). Merging reflective inquiry and self-study as a framework for enhancing the scholarship of teaching. *Journal of Nursing Education, 41*(9), 413–418.

Duchscher, J. B. (2004). Transition to professional nursing practice: Emerging issues and initiatives. In M. Oermann & K. Heinrich (Eds.), *Annual review of nursing education* (Vol. II, pp. 283–303). New York: Springer Publishing.

Elbow, P. (1997). High stakes and low stakes in assigning and responding to writing. *New Directions for Teaching and Learning, 69*, 5–13.

Ellerton, M-L., & Gregor, F. (2003). A study of transition: The new nurse graduate at 3 months. *Journal of Continuing Education in Nursing, 34*(3), 103–107.

Farella, C. (2002). School of hard knocks: Is racism a fixture of nursing academia? *Nursing Spectrum, 14*(12), 34–35.

Ferguson, L. (2004). External validity, generalizability, and knowledge utilization. *Journal of Nursing Scholarship, 36*(1), 16–22.

Ferketich, S. (1991). Aspects of item analysis. *Research in Nursing and Health, 14,* 165–168.

Flege, J. E., & Liu, S. (2001). The effects of experience on adults' acquisition of a second language. *Studies in Second Language Acquisition, 23*(4), 527–552.

Foley, R., & Wurmser, T. A. (2004). Culture diversity: A mobile workforce command creative leadership, new partnerships, and innovative approaches to integration. *Nursing Administration Quarterly, 28*(2), 122–128.

Fortier, J. P., & Bishop, D. (2003). *Setting the agenda for research on cultural competence in health care: Final report.* Rockville, MD: U.S. Department of Health and Human Services Office of Minority Health and Agency for Healthcare Research and Quality.

Fuertes, J. N., & Westbrook, F. D. (1996). Using the social, attitudinal, familial, and environmental (S.A.F.E.) acculturation stress scale to assess the adjustment needs of Hispanic college students. *Measurement and Evaluation in Counseling and Development, 29,* 67–76.

Gaffney, K. F. (2000). Encouraging collaborative learning among culturally diverse students. *Nurse Educator, 25*(5), 219–221.

Georges, C. A. (2004). African American nurse leadership: Pathways and opportunities. *Nursing Administration Quarterly, 28*(3), 170–172.

Giger, J., & Davidhizar, R. (1999). *Transcultural nursing: Assessment and intervention* (3rd ed.). St. Louis, MO: Mosby.

Gigliotti, E. (1999). Women's multiple role stress: Testing Neuman's flexible line of defense. *Nursing Science Quarterly, 12*(1), 36–44.

Gigliotti, E. (2001). Development of the perceived multiple role stress scale (PMRS). *Journal of Nursing Measurement, 9*(2), 163–180.

Gilley, W. F., & Uhlig, G. E. (1993). Factor analysis and ordinal data. *Education, 114,* 258–264.

Gist, M. E., & Mitchell, T. R. (1992). Self-efficacy: A theoretical analysis of its determinants and malleability. *Academy of Management Review, 17,* 183–211.

Gloria, A. M., & Kurpius, S. E. R. (1996). The validation of the cultural congruity scale and the university environment scale with Chicano/a students. *Hispanic Journal of Behavioral Sciences, 18*(4), 533–549.

Gomez, G. E., & White, M. J. (2002). An international educational experience. *Hispanic Health Care International, 1*(3), 124–127.

Greenhaus, J. H., & Beutell, N. J. (1985). Sources of conflict between work and family roles. *Academy of Management Review, 10,* 76–88.

Griffiths, M. J., & Tagliareni, M. E. (1999). Challenging traditional assumptions about minority students in nursing education. *Nursing & Health Care Perspectives, 20,* 290–295.

Hackett, G. (1985). Role of mathematics self-efficacy in the choice of math-related majors of college women and men: A path analysis. *Journal of Counseling Psychology, 32*(1), 47–56.

Hall, C. C. I. (1992). Coloring outside the lines. In M. P. P. Root (Ed.), *Racially mixed people in America* (pp. 326–329). Newbury Park, CA: Sage.

Haloburdo, E. P., & Thompson, M. A. (1998). A comparison of international learning experiences for baccalaureate nursing students: Developed and developing countries. *Journal of Nursing Education, 37*(1), 13–21.

Harden, J. K. (2003). Faculty and student experiences with web-based discussion groups in a large lecture setting. *Nurse Educator, 28*(1), 26–30.

Harrington, S. S., & Walker, B. L. (2004). The effects of computer-based training on immediate and residual learning of nursing facility staff. *Journal of Continuing Education in Nursing, 35*(4), 154–163.

Harrow, A. J. (1972). *A taxonomy of the psychomotor domain: A guide for developing behavioral objectives* . New York: McKay.

Heller, B. R., Drenkard, K., Esposito-Herr, M. B., Romano, C., Tom, S., & Valentine, N. (2004). Educating nurses for leadership roles. *Journal of Continuing Education in Nursing, 35*(5), 203–210.

Heller, B. R., Oros, M. T., & Durney-Crowley, J. (2000). The future of nursing education: 10 trends to watch. *Nursing and Health Care Perspectives, 21*(1), 9–13.

Huff, C. (1997). Cooperative learning: A model for teaching. *Journal of Nursing Education, 36*(9), 434–436.

International Council of Nurses (ICN). (1973). *Code for nurses.* Geneva, Switzerland: Author.

Jalili-Grenier, F., & Chase, M. M. (1997). Retention of nursing students with English as a second language. *Journal of Advanced Nursing, 25*, 199–203.

Jeffreys, M. R. (1991). Time out! Let's play charades. *Nurse Educator, 16*(5), 12, 34.

Jeffreys, M. R. (1993). *The relationship of self-efficacy and select academic and environmental variables on academic achievement and retention.* Unpublished doctoral dissertation, Teachers College, Columbia University, New York, NY.

Jeffreys, M. R. (1994). *Transcultural Self-Efficacy Tool (TSET).* Unpublished instrument, copyrighted by author.

Jeffreys, M. R. (2000). Development and psychometric evaluation of the Transcultural Self-Efficacy Tool: A synthesis of findings. *Journal of Transcultural Nursing, 11*(2), 127–136.

Jeffreys, M. R. (2002). A transcultural core course in the clinical nurse specialist curriculum. *Clinical Nurse Specialist: The Journal for Advanced Nursing Practice.* 16(4), 195–202.

Jeffreys, M. R. (2004). *Nursing student retention: Understanding the process and making a difference.* New York: Springer Publishing.

Jeffreys, M. R. (2005a). Raising awareness: A quest for new directions in cultural competence development. *Journal of Multicultural Nursing and Health, 11*(2), 5–6.

Jeffreys, M. R. (2005b). Clinical nurse specialists as cultural brokers, change agents, and partners in meeting the needs of culturally diverse populations. *Journal of Multicultural Nursing and Health, 11*(2), 41–48.

Jeffreys, M. R. (2006). Cultural competence in clinical practice. *NSNA Imprint,* *53*(2), 37–41.

Jeffreys, M. R., Massoni, M., O'Donnell, M., & Smodlaka, I. (1997). Student evaluation of courses: Determining the reliability and validity of three survey instruments. *Journal of Nursing Education, 36*(8), 397–400.

Jeffreys, M. R., & O'Donnell M. (1997). Cultural discovery: An innovative philosophy for creative learning activities. *Journal of Transcultural Nursing, 8*(2), 17–22.

Jeffreys, M. R., & Smodlaka, I. (1996). Steps of the instrument-design process: An illustrative approach for nurse educators. *Nurse Educator, 21*(6), 47–52 [Erratum 1997, 22(1), 49].

Jeffreys, M. R., & Smodlaka, I. (1998). Exploring the factorial composition of the Transcultural Self-Efficacy Tool. *International Journal of Nursing Studies, 35*, 217–225.

Jeffreys, M. R., & Smodlaka, I. (1999a). Changes in students' transcultural self-efficacy perceptions following an integrated approach to culture care. *Journal of Multicultural Nursing and Health, 5*(2), 6–12 [Erratum 2000, 6(1), 20].

Jeffreys, M. R., & Smodlaka, I. (1999b). Construct validation of the Transcultural Self-Efficacy Tool. *Journal of Nursing Education, 38*, 222–227.

Jeffreys, M. R., & Zoucha, R. (2001). The invisible culture of the multiracial, multiethnic individual: A transcultural imperative. *Journal of Cultural Diversity, 8*(3), 79–83.

Joel, L. A., & Kelly, L. Y. (2002). *The nursing experience: Trends, challenges, and transitions.* New York: McGraw-Hill.

Johnson, T. P., Jobe, J. B., O'Rourke, D., Sudman, S., Warnecke, R. B., Chávez, N., et al. (1997). Dimensions of self-identification among multiracial and multiethnic respondents in survey interviews. *Evaluation Review, 21*(6), 671–687.

Joint Commission on Accreditation of Healthcare Organizations (JCAHO). (2002). *Health care at the crossroads: Strategies for addressing the evolving nursing crisis.* Washington, DC: Author.

Jones-Schenk, J., & Yoder-Wise, P. S. (2002). Professional self-regulation: Another Enron casualty? *Journal of Continuing Education in Nursing, 33*(3), 100–101.

Kataoka-Yahiro, M. R., & Abriam-Yago, K. (1997). Culturally competent teaching strategies for Asian nursing students for whom English is a second language. *Journal of Cultural Diversity, 4*(3), 83–87.

Kavanagh, K. H., & Kennedy, P. H. (1992). *Promoting cultural diversity: Strategies for health care.* Newbury Park, CA: Sage.

Keane, M. (1993). Preferred learning styles and study strategies in a linguistically diverse baccalaureate nursing student population. *Journal of Nursing Education, 32*(5), 214–221.

Kelly, E. (1997). Development of strategies to identify the learning needs of baccalaureate nursing students. *Journal of Nursing Education, 36*, 156–162.

Keltner, B., Kelley, F. J., & Smith, D. (2004). Leadership to reduce health disparities: A model for nursing leadership in American Indian communities. *Nursing Administration Quarterly, 28*(3), 181–190.

Khoiny, F. E. (1995). Factors that contribute to computer-assisted instruction effectiveness. *Computers in Nursing, 13*(4), 165–168.

Kim, J., & Mueller, C. W. (1978). *Factor analysis: Statistical methods and practical issues.* Newbury Park, CA: Sage.

Kimball, B., & O'Neil, E. (2002). *Health care's human crisis: The American nursing shortage.* Princeton, NJ: Robert Wood Johnson.

Kirkland, M. L. S. (1998). Stressors and coping strategies among successful female African American baccalaureate nursing students. *Journal of Nursing Education, 37*(1), 5–12.

Knapp, T. R. (1990). Treating ordinal scales as interval scales: An attempt to resolve the controversy. *Nursing Research, 39*(2), 121–123.

Knapp, T. R. (1993). Treating ordinal scales as ordinal scales. *Nursing Research, 42*(3), 184–186.

Koeckeritz, J., Malkiewicz, J., & Henderson, A. (2002). The seven principles of good practice: Applications for online education in nursing. *Nurse Educator, 27*(6), 283–287.

Koenig, J. M., & Zorn, C. R. (2002). Using storytelling as an approach to teaching and learning with diverse students. *Journal of Nursing Education, 41*(9), 393–399.

Kollar, S. J., & Ailinger, R. L. (2002). International clinical experiences: Long-term impact on students. *Nurse Educator, 27*(1), 28–31.

Kramer, N. (1995). Using games for learning. *Journal of Continuing Education in Nursing, 26*, 40–42.

Knowles, M. (1984). *The adult learner: A neglected species.* Houston, TX: Gulf.

Krathwohl, D. R., Bloom, B. S., & Masia, B. (Eds.). (1964). *Taxonomy of educational objectives: Handbook II: Affective domain.* New York: McKay.

Kubsch, S., Henniges, A., Lorenzoni, N., Eckardt, S., & Oleniczak, S. (2003). Factors influencing accruement of contact hours for nurses. *Journal of Continuing Education in Nursing, 34*(5), 205–212.

Kurz, J. M. (1993). The adult ESL baccalaureate nursing student. *Journal of Nursing Education, 32*(5), 227–229.

Labun, E. (2002). The Red River College model: Enhancing success for native Canadian and other nursing students from disenfranchised groups. *Journal of Transcultural Nursing, 13*(4), 311–317.

Lambert, V. A., & Nugent, K. E. (1994). Addressing the academic progression of students encountering mental health problems. *Nurse Educator, 19*(5), 33–39.

Lee, C., & Bobko, P. (1994). Self-efficacy beliefs: Comparison of five measures. *Journal of Applied Psychology, 79*(3), 364–369.

Lee, S. M., & Fernandez, M. (1998). Trends in Asian American racial/ethnic intermarriage: A comparison of 1980 and 1990 census data. *Sociological Perspectives, 41*(2), 323–342.

Leininger, M. M. (1989). Transcultural nurse specialists and generalists: New practitioners in nursing. *Journal of Transcultural Nursing, 1*, 4–16.

Leininger, M. M. (1991a). *Culture care diversity and universality: A theory of nursing.* New York: National League for Nursing.

Leininger, M. M. (1991b). Transcultural care principles, human rights, and ethical considerations. *Journal of Transcultural Nursing, 3*(1), 21–23.

Leininger, M. M. (1991c). Leininger's acculturation health care assessment guide for cultural patterns in traditional & non-traditional life ways. *Journal of Transcultural Nursing, 2*(2), 40–42.

Leininger, M. M. (1994a). *Transcultural nursing: Concepts, theories, and practices.* Columbus, OH: Greyden Press.

Leininger, M. M. (1994b). Are nurses prepared to function worldwide? *Journal of Transcultural Nursing, 5*(2), 2–4.

Leininger, M. M. (1995a). *Transcultural nursing: Concepts, theories, research, and practice.* Blacklick, OH: McGraw-Hill College Custom Services.

Leininger, M. M. (1995b). Teaching transcultural nursing in undergraduate and graduate programs. *Journal of Transcultural Nursing, 6*(2), 10–26.

Leininger, M. M. (2002a). Essential transcultural nursing care concepts, principles, examples, and policy statements. In M. M. Leininger & M. R. McFarland (Eds.), *Transcultural nursing: Concepts, theories, research, and practice* (3rd ed., pp. 45–69). New York: McGraw-Hill.

Leininger, M. M. (2002b). The future of transcultural nursing: A global perspective. In M. M. Leininger & M. R. McFarland (Eds.), *Transcultural nursing: Concepts, theories, research, and practice* (3rd ed., pp. 585–58). New York: McGraw-Hill.

Leininger, M. M. (2002c). Part I. The Theory of culture care and the ethnonursing research method. In M. M. Leininger & M.R. McFarland (2002). *Transcultural nursing: Concepts, theories, research, & practice* (3rd ed., pp. 71–98). New York: McGraw-Hill.

Leininger, M. M., & McFarland, M. R. (2002). *Transcultural nursing: Concepts, theories, research, and practice* (3rd ed.). New York: McGraw-Hill.

Lent, R. W., Brown, S. D., & Gore, P. A. (1997). Discriminant and predictive validity of academic self-concept, academic self-efficacy, and mathematics-specific self-efficacy. *Journal of Counseling Psychology, 44*(3), 307–315.

Lent, R. W., Brown, S. D., & Larkin, K. C. (1986). Self-efficacy in prediction of academic performance and career options. *Journal of Counseling Psychology, 33*(3), 265–269.

Lent, R. W., Brown, S. D., & Larkin, K. C. (1987). Comparison of three theoretically derived variables in predicting career and academic behavior: Self-efficacy, interest congruence, and consequence thinking. *Journal of Counseling Psychology, 34*(3), 293–298.

Lent, R. W., Lopez, F. G., & Bieschke, K. J. (1993). Predicting mathematics-related choice and success behaviors: Test of an expanded social cognitive model. *Journal of Vocational Behavior, 42,* 223–236.

Lim, J., Downie, J., & Nathan, P. (2004). Nursing students' self-efficacy in providing transcultural care. *Nurse Education Today, 24*(6), 428–234.

LoBiondo-Wood, G., & Haber, J. (1998). *Nursing research: Methods, critical appraisal, and utilization* (4th ed.). New York: Mosby.

Loerch, K. J., Russell, J. E. A., & Rush, M. C. (1989). The relationships among family domain variables and work–family conflict for men and women. *Journal of Vocational Behavior, 35,* 288–308.

MacIntosh, J., MacKay, E., Mallet-Boucher, M., & Wiggins, N. (2002). Discovering co-learning with students in distance education sites. *Nurse Educator, 27*(4), 182–186.

MacQuarrie, D. (2004). *Assessment of student nurses' transcultural self-efficacy perceptions (confidence) when caring for culturally diverse clients.* Unpublished doctoral dissertation, McMaster University, Hamilton, Ontario, Canada.

Maddux, J. E. (1995). *Self-efficacy, adaptation, and adjustment: Theory, research, and application.* New York: Plenum Press.

Madorin, S., & Iwasiw, C. (1999). The effects of computer-assisted instruction on the self-efficacy of baccalaureate nursing students. *Journal of Nursing Education, 38*(6), 282–285.

Management Sciences for Health (MSH). (2005). *Providers guide to quality and culture.* Retrieved January 30, 2005, from http://www.msh.org/programs_guide.html.

Manifold, C., & Rambur, B. (2001). Predictors of attrition in American Indian nursing students. *Journal of Nursing Education, 40*(6), 279–281.

Mateo, M. A., & McMyler, E. (2004). The nurse educator role in staff competency. In M. Oermann & K. Heinrich (Eds.), *Annual review of nursing education* (Vol. II, pp. 305–325). New York: Springer Publishing.

Mathews, M. B. (2003). Resourcing nursing education through collaboration. *Journal of Continuing Education in Nursing, 34*(6), 251–257.

Matzo, M. L., Sherman, D. W., Mazanec, P., Barber, M. A., Virani, R., & McLaughlin, M. M. (2002). Teaching cultural considerations at the end of life: End of life nursing education consortium program recommendations. *Journal of Continuing Education in Nursing, 33*(6), 270–278.

Maville, J., & Huerta, C. G. (1997). Stress and social support among Hispanic student nurses: Implications for academic achievement. *Journal of Cultural Diversity, 4*(1), 18–25.

Medley, C. F., & Horne, C. (2005). Using simulation technology for undergraduate nursing education. *Journal of Nursing Education, 44*(1), 31–34.

Mertig, R. G. (2003). *Teaching nursing in an associate degree program.* New York: Springer.

Miller, J. (1997). Politics and care: A study of Czech Americans within Leininger's theory of culture care diversity and universality. *Journal of Transcultural Nursing, 9*(1), 3–13.

Miller, J., Koyanagi, M. L. S., & Morgan, K. J. (2005). Faculty as a community engaged with ongoing curricular development: Use of groupware and electronic resources. *Journal of Nursing Education, 44*(1), 27–30.

Moch, S. D., Long, G. L., Jones, J. W., Shadlick, K., & Solheim, K. (1999). Faculty and student cross-cultural learning through teaching health promotion in the community. *Journal of Nursing Education, 38*(5), 238–240.

Mone, M. A., Baker, D. D., & Jeffries, F. (1995). Predictive validity and time dependency of self-efficacy, self-esteem, personal goals, and academic performance. *Educational and Psychological Measurement, 55*(5), 716–727.

Morton, P. G., & Rauen, C. A. (2004). Using simulation in nursing education: The University of Maryland and Georgetown University experiences. In M. Oermann & K. Heinrich (Eds.), *Annual review of nursing education* (Vol. II, pp. 139–161). New York: Springer Publishing.

Mueller, S. S., Pullen, R. L., & McGee, K. S. (2002). A model nursing computer resource center. *Nurse Educator, 27*(3), 115–117.

Multon, K. D., Brown, S. D., & Lent, R. W. (1991). Relation of self-efficacy beliefs to academic outcomes: A meta-analytic investigation. *Journal of Counseling Psychology, 38*(1), 30–38.

Munro, B. H. (2005). *Statistical methods for health care research* (5th ed.). New York: Lippincott Williams & Wilkins.

Nash, G. B. (1995). The hidden history of mestizo in America. *Journal of American History, 82*(3), 941–962.

National League for Nursing (NLN). (2002a). *Nursing Education Research, Technology and Information Management Advisory Council (NER-TIMAC)*. Retrieved April 2, 2003, from http://www.nln.org/aboutnln/nertimac.htm.

National League for Nursing (NLN). (2002b). *Priorities for research in nursing education*. Retrieved April 2, 2003, from http://www.nln.org/aboutnln/research.htm.

Nehring, W. M., & Lashley, F. R. (2004). Using the human patient simulator in nursing education. In M. Oermann & K. Heinrich (Eds.), *Annual review of nursing education* (Vol. II, pp. 163–181). New York: Springer Publishing.

Nunnally, J. C., & Bernstein, I. H. (1994). *Psychometric theory*. New York: McGraw-Hill.

Nurmi, J-E., & Aunola, K. (2001). How does academic achievement come about: Cross-cultural and methodological notes. *International Journal of Educational Research, 35*, 403–409.

Oermann, M. H., & Gaberson, K. B. (1998). *Evaluation and testing in nursing education*. New York: Springer Publishing.

Office of Minority Health (OMH). (2001). *National standards for culturally and linguistically appropriate services in health care*. Washington, DC: U.S. Department of Health and Human Services.

Office of Minority Health (OMH). (2005). *Attachment 3: Potential measures/indicators of cultural competence*. Retrieved January 30, 2005, from http://www.hrsa.gov/OMH/cultural/attachment3.htm.

Olenchak, F. R., & Hebert, T. P. (2002). Endangered academic talent: Lessons learned from gifted first-generation college males. *Journal of College Student Development, 43*(2), 195–212.

Ostrow, L., & DiMaria-Ghalili, R. A. (2005). Distance education for graduate nursing: One state school's experience. *Journal of Nursing Education, 44*(1), 5–10.

Pacquiao, D. (2004). Building collaborative influence. *Journal of Transcultural Nursing, 15*(2), 155.

Pascoe, P. (1996). Miscegenation law, court cases, and ideologies of "race" in twentieth-century America. *Journal of American History, 83*(1), 44–69.

Pastuszak, J., & Rodowicz, M. O. (2002). Internal e-mail: An avenue of education opportunity. *Journal of Continuing Education in Nursing, 33*(4), 164–167.

Patterson, B. J., & Morin, K. H. (2002). Perceptions of the maternal-child clinical rotation: The male student nurse experience. *Journal of Nursing Education, 41*(6), 266–272.

Perlmann, J. (1997). Multiracials, intermarriage, and ethnicity. *Society, 6,* 20–23.

Pickerell, K. D. (2001). A cross-cultural nursing experience on the Rosebud reservation. *Nurse Educator, 26*(3), 128–131.

Piercy, E. C. (2004). Using WebQuests to promote active learning. *Journal of Continuing Education in Nursing, 35*(5), 200–201.

Pimple, C., Schmidt, L., & Tidwell, S. (2003). Achieving excellence in end-of-life care. *Nurse Educator, 28*(1), 40–43.

Pinderhughes, E. (1995). Biracial identity—Asset or handicap? In H. W. Harris, C. Blue, & E. E. H. Griffith (Eds.), *Racial and ethnic identity: Psychological development and creative expression* (pp. 73–93). New York: Routledge.

Pinkerton, S. E. (2004). The financial return on education programs. *Journal of Continuing Education in Nursing, 35*(6), 244–245.

Pintrich, P. R., & Garcia, T. (1994). Self-regulated learning in college students: Knowledge, strategies, and motivation. In P. R. Pintrich, D. R. Brown, & C. E. Weinstein (Eds.), *Student motivation, cognition, and learning: Essays in honor of Wilbert J. McKeachie* (pp. 113–133). Hillsdale, NJ: Erlbaum.

Platter, B. (2005, October). *Clinical nurse cultural competency pre and post transcultural nursing education.* Paper presented at the annual conference of the Transcultural Nursing Society, New York, NY.

Polit, D. F., & Beck, C. T. (2004). *Nursing research: Principles and methods.* New York: Lippincott Williams & Wilkins.

Porter, C. P., & Barbee, E. (2004). Race and racism in nursing research: Past, present, and future. In L. Fitzpatrick (Ed.), *Annual review of nursing research* (Vol. 22, pp. 9–38). New York: Springer Publishing.

Pullen, R. L., Murray, P. H., & McGee, K. S. (2001). Care groups: A model to mentor novice nursing students. *Nurse Educator, 26,* 283–288.

Pullen, R. L., Murray, P. H., & McGee, K. S. (2003). Using care groups to mentor novice nursing students. In M. Oermann & K. Heinrich (Eds.), *Annual review of nursing education* (Vol. I, pp. 147–161). New York: Springer Publishing.

Purnell, L. D. (2003). Purnell's model for cultural competence. In L. D. Purnell & B. J. Paulanka (Eds.), *Transcultural health care: A culturally competent approach* (2nd ed., pp. 8–39). Philadelphia: FA Davis.

Purnell, L. D., & Paulanka, B. J. (2003). *Transcultural health care: A culturally competent approach* (2nd ed.). Philadelphia: FA Davis.

Ransdell, S. (2001a). Predicting college success: The importance of ability and non-cognitive variables. *International Journal of Educational Research, 35,* 357–364.

Ransdell, S. (2001b). Discussion and implications. *International Journal of Educational Research, 35,* 391–395.

Ransdell, S., Hawkins, C., & Adams, R. (2001a). Models, modeling, and the design of the study. *International Journal of Educational Research, 35*, 365–372.

Ransdell, S., Hawkins, C., & Adams, R. (2001b). Results of the study. *International Journal of Educational Research, 35*, 373–389.

Rashotte, J., & Thomas, M. (2002). Incorporating educational theory into critical care orientation. *Journal of Continuing Education in Nursing, 33*(3), 131–137.

Rauen, C. (2001). Using simulation to teach critical thinking skills: You can't just throw the book at them. *Critical Care Nursing Clinics of North America, 13*, 93–103.

Rendon, L. I. (1994). Validating culturally diverse students: Toward a new model of learning & student development. *Innovative Higher Education, 19*(1), 23–32.

Rendon, L. I., Jalomo, R. E., & Nora, A. (2000). Theoretical considerations in the study of minority student retention in higher education. In J. M. Braxton (Ed.), *Reworking the student departure puzzle* (pp. 127–156). Nashville, TN: Vanderbilt University Press.

Rew, L. (1996). Affirming cultural diversity: A pathways model for nursing faculty. *Journal of Nursing Education, 35*(7), 310–314.

Riley, J. M., Beal, J., Levi, P., & McCausland, M. P. (2002). Revisioning nursing scholarship. *Journal of Nursing Scholarship, 34*(4), 383–389.

Rizzolo, M. A. (2002). Where have all the teachers gone? Long time passing. . . . *Shaping the Future, 1*(1), 2–4.

Root, M. P. P. (1992). Within, between, and beyond race. In M. P. P. Root (Ed.), *Racially mixed people in America* (pp. 3–11). Newbury Park, CA: Sage.

Root, M. P. P. (1997). Multiracial Asians: Models of ethnic identity. *Ameriasia Journal, 23*(1), 29–41.

Ryan, M., Twibell, R., Brigham, C., & Bennett, P. (2000). Learning to care for clients in their world, not mine. *Journal of Nursing Education, 39*(9), 401–408.

Saks, A. M. (1995). Longitudinal field investigation of the moderating and mediating effects of self-efficacy on the relationship between training and newcomer adjustment. *Journal of Applied Psychology, 80*, 211–225.

Sands, N., & Schuh, J. H. (2004). Identifying interventions to improve the retention of biracial students: A case study. *Journal of College Student Retention: Research, Theory, and Practice, 5*(4), 349–363.

Schmidt, L. A. (2004a). Psychometric evaluation of the writing-to-learn attitude survey. *Journal of Nursing Education, 43*(10), 458–465.

Schmidt, L. A. (2004b). Evaluating the writing-to-learn strategy with undergraduate nursing students. *Journal of Nursing Education, 43*(10), 466–473.

Schön, D. (1987). *Educating the reflective practitioner.* San Francisco: Jossey-Bass.

Schoolcraft, V., & Novotny, J. (2000). *A nuts and bolts approach to teaching nursing.* New York: Springer Publishing.

Schunk, D. (1987). *Self-efficacy and cognitive achievement.* Paper presented at the annual meeting of the American Psychological Association, New York, NY. (ERIC Document Reproduction Service No. ED 287 880).

Schunk, D. (1995). Self-efficacy and education and instruction. In J. E. Maddux (Ed.), *Self-efficacy, adaptation, and adjustment: Theory, research, and application* (pp. 281–304). New York: Plenum.

Shell, D. F., Murphy, C. C., & Bruning, R. H. (1989). Self-efficacy and outcome expectancy mechanisms in reading and writing achievement. *Journal of Educational Psychology, 81,* 91–100.

Shinn, L. J. (1998). Contemporary issues in professional organizations. In D. J. Mason & J. K. Leavitt, (Eds.), *Policy and politics in nursing and health care* (3rd ed., p. 525–534). New York: WB Saunders.

Simpson, R. L. (2004). Recruit, retain, assess: Technology's role in diversity. *Nursing Administration Quarterly, 28*(3), 217–220.

Skaggs, B. J., & DeVries, C. M. (1998). You and your professional organization. In D. J. Mason & J. K. Leavitt, (Ed.), *Policy and politics in nursing and health care* (3rd ed, pp. 535–545). New York: WB Saunders.

Smart, J. F., & Smart, D.W. (1995). Acculturative stress: The experience of the Hispanic immigrant. *The Counseling Psychologist, 23,* 25–42.

Sommer, S. (2001). Multicultural nursing education. *Journal of Nursing Education, 40*(6), 276–278.

Spector, R. E. (2004). *Cultural diversity in health and illness* (6th ed.). Upper Saddle River, NJ: Pearson/Prentice Hall.

Spickard, P. R. (1997). What must I be? Asian Americans and the question of multiethnic identity. *Ameriasia Journal, 23*(1), 43–60.

Spickard, P. R., & Fong, R. (1995). Pacific Islander Americans and the question of multiethnicity: A vision of America's future? *Social Forces, 73*(4), 1365–1383.

Squires, A. (2002). New graduate orientation in the rural community hospital. *Journal of Continuing Education in Nursing, 33*(5), 203–209.

St. Clair, A., & McKenry, L. (1999). Preparing culturally competent practitioners. *Journal of Nursing Education, 38*(5), 228–234.

St. Hill, P., Lipson, J. G., & Meleis, A. I. (2003). *Caring for women cross-culturally.* Philadelphia: Davis.

Stage, F. K., & Hossler, D. (2000). Where is the student? Linking student behaviors, college choice, and college persistence. In J. Braxton (Ed.), *Reworking the student departure puzzle* (pp. 170–195). Nashville, TN: Vanderbilt University.

Sternberger, C. S. (2002). Embedding a pedagogical model in the design of an online course. *Nurse Educator, 27*(4), 170–173.

Stevens, G. L. (1998). Experience the culture. *Journal of Nursing Education, 37*(1), 30–33.

Stevenson, E. L. (2003). Future trends in nursing employment. *American Journal of Nursing Career Guide, 2003,* 19–25.

Stigler, J. W., & Hiebert, J. (1998). Teaching is a cultural activity. *American Educator, Winter,* 4–11.

Storch, J., & Gamroth, L. (2002). Scholarship revisited: A collaborative nursing education program's journey. *Journal of Nursing Education, 41*(12), 524–530.

Streubert, H. J. (1994). Male nursing students' perceptions of clinical experience. *Nurse Educator, 19*(5), 28–32.

Sudman, S., & Bradburn, N. M. (1991). *Asking questions.* San Francisco: Jossey-Bass.

Swanson, J. W. (2004). Diversity: Creating an environment of inclusiveness. *Nursing Education Quarterly, 28*(3), 207–211.

Tabi, M. M., & Mukherjee, S. (2003). Nursing in a global community: A study abroad program. *Journal of Transcultural Nursing, 14*(2), 134–138.

Tanner, C. A. (2002). Learning to teach: An introduction to "Teacher Talk: New Pedagogies for Nursing." *Journal of Nursing Education, 41*(3), 95–96.

Tayebi, K., Moore-Jazayeri, M., & Maynard, T. (1998). From the borders: Reforming the curriculum for the at-risk student. *Journal of Cultural Diversity, 5*(3), 101–109.

Thede, L. Q., Taft, S., & Coeling, H. (1994). Computer-assisted instruction: A learner's viewpoint. *Journal of Nursing Education, 33*(7), 299–305.

Thompson, P. A. (2004). Leadership from an international perspective. *Nursing Administration Quarterly, 28*(3), 191–198.

Thorpe, K., & Loo, R. (2003). The values profile of nursing undergraduate students: Implications for education and professional development. *Journal of Nursing Education, 42*(2), 83–90.

Tomey, A. M. (2003). Learning with cases. *Journal of Continuing Education in Nursing, 34*(1), 34–38.

Toney, D. (2004). *Exploring the relationship between levels of cultural competence and the perceived level of quality care among registered nurses caring for culturally diverse patients.* Unpublished doctoral dissertation, Capella University. Minneapolis, MN.

Tucker-Allen, S., & Long, E. (1999). *Recruitment and retention of minority students: Stories of success.* Lisle, IL: Tucker Publications.

Ulrich, D. L., & Glendon, K. J. (1999). *Interactive group learning: Strategies for nurse educators.* New York: Springer Publishing.

Upton, T. A., & Lee-Thompson, L-C. (2001). The role of the first language in second language reading. *Studies in Second Language Acquisition, 23*(4), 469–495.

U.S. Census Bureau. (2002). *United States Census 2000.* Retrieved February 17, 2006, from http://www.census.gov/main/www/cen2000.html.

Vance, C., & Olson, R. K. (1998). *The mentor connection in nursing.* New York: Springer.

Velez, J. (2005). *The effects of cultural competency training using self-instruction on obstetrical nurses' awareness, knowledge, and attitudes.* Unpublished master's thesis, Cleveland State University, Cleveland, OH.

Villarruel, A. M., & Peragallo, N. (2004). Leadership development of Hispanic nurses. *Nursing Administration Quarterly, 28*(3), 173–180.

Villaruel, A. M., Canales, M., & Torres, S. (2001). Bridges and barriers: Educational mobility of Hispanic nurses. *Journal of Nursing Education, 40*(6), 245–251.

Waltz, C. F., Strickland, O. L., & Lenz, E. R. (2005). *Measurement in nursing research.* Philadelphia: Davis.

Washington, D., Erickson, J. I., & Ditomassi, M. (2004). Mentoring the minority leader of tomorrow. *Nursing Administration Quarterly, 28*(3), 165–169.

Weaver, H. N. (2001). Indigenous nurses and professional education: Friends or foes? *Journal of Nursing Education, 40*(6), 252–258.

Weis, P. A., & Guyton-Simmons, J. (1998). A computer simulation for teaching critical thinking. *Nurse Educator, 23*(2), 30–33.

White, M. J., Amos, E., & Kouzekanani, K. (1999). Problem-based learning: An outcomes student. *Nurse Educator, 24*(2), 33–36.

Williams, M. E., & Jones, J. J. (2004). Creating staff-friendly continuing education: The tidbits and niblets program. *Journal of Continuing Education in Nursing, 35*(6), 248–249.

Williams, R. P., & Calvillo, E. R. (2002). Maximizing learning among students from culturally diverse backgrounds. *Nurse Educator, 27*(5), 222–226.

Wilson, L., & Houghtaling, S. (2001). *Report on a study of cultural competence teaching in California medical and dental schools.* Retrieved February 15, 2006, from http://www.dca.ca.gov/cltaskforce/appendix_f.pdf# search='Report%20on%20a%20study%20of%20cultural%20competence %20 teaching% 20in% 20 California% 20medical% 20and% 20dental%20 schools'.

Winters, C., & Owens, R. (1993). Alternative teaching strategies: Using a health fair to meet tribal college and nursing program needs. *Journal of Nursing Education, 32*(5), 237–238.

Xiao, J. (2005). Resources in transcultural nursing: A library orientation program for nursing students. *Journal of Multicultural Nursing and Health, 11*(2), 56–63.

Yoder, M. K. (1996). Instructional responses to ethnically diverse nursing students. *Journal of Nursing Education, 35*(7), 315–321.

Yoder, M. K. (2001). The bridging approach: Effective strategies for teaching ethnically diverse nursing students. *Journal of Transcultural Nursing, 12*, 319–325.

Yoder, M. K., & Saylor, C. (2002). Student and teacher roles: Mismatched expectations. *Nurse Educator, 27*(5), 201–203.

Young, P., & Diekelmann, N. (2002). Learning to lecture: Exploring the skills, strategies, and practices of new teachers in nursing education. *Journal of Nursing Education, 41*(9), 405–412.

Yurkovich, E. E. (2001). Working with American Indians toward educational success. *Journal of Nursing Education, 40*(6), 259–269.

Zimmerman, B. J. (1995). Self-efficacy and educational development. In A. Bandura (Ed.), *Self-efficacy in changing societies* (pp. 202–231). New York: Cambridge University Press.

Zimmerman, B. J. (1996). Enhancing student academic and health functioning: A self-regulatory perspective. *School Psychology Quarterly, 11*(1), 47–66.

Zinatelli, M., Dube, M. A., & Jovanovic, R. (2002). Computer-based study skills training: The role of technology in improving performance and retention. *Journal of College Student Retention: Research, Theory, & Practice, 4*(1), 67–78.

Index

Page numbers followed by *f* indicate figure; those followed by *t* indicate table; those followed by *b* indicate box.

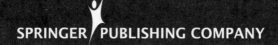

SPRINGER PUBLISHING COMPANY

Self-Efficacy in Nursing
Research and Measurement Perspectives

Elizabeth R. Lenz, PhD, FAAN
Lillie M. Shortridge-Baggett, EdD, RN, FAAN, Editors

Self-efficacy, or the belief that one can self-manage one's own health, is an important goal of health care providers, particularly in chronic illness. This book explores the concept of self-efficacy from theory, research, measurement, and practice perspectives. The core of the book is an international collaboration of nurses from the U.S. and the Netherlands who have developed tools for promoting and measuring self-efficacy in diabetes management. Originally developed as a special issue of the journal *Scholarly Inquiry for Nursing Practice,* the book addresses the importance of theory-based interventions in enhancing self-efficacy.

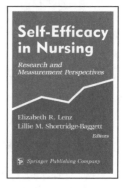

Partial Contents:

Part I: Introduction

- Self-Efficacy: Measurement and Intervention in Nursing
  L.M. Shortridge-Baggett
- The Theory and Measurement of the Self-Efficacy Construct
  J.J. van der Bijl and L.M. Shortridge-Baggett

Part II: Self-Efficacy in Diabetes Management

- Self-Efficacy in Children with Diabetes Mellitus: Testing of a Measurement
  Instrument, *M.J. Kappen, et al.*
- Strategies Enhancing Self-Efficacy in Diabetes Education: A Review
  K.E.W. van der Laar and *J.J. van der Bijl*

Part III: Self-Efficacy and Other Clinical Conditions

- Self-Efficacy Targeted Treatments for Weight Loss in
  Postmenopausal Women, *K.E. Dennis, et al.*
- An Intervention to Increase Quality of Life and Self-Care Self-Efficacy and
  Decrease Symptoms in Breast Cancer Patients, *E.L. Lev, et al.*

2002 · 128pp · 0-8261-1563-2 · hardcover

11 West 42nd Street, New York, NY 10036-8002 • Fax: 212-941-7842
Order Toll-Free: 877-687-7476 • Order On-line: www.springerpub.com

Teaching Evidence-Based Practice in Nursing

Rona F. Levin, PhD, RN
Harriet R. Feldman, PhD, RN, FAAN, Editors

"In their outstanding book, Rona Levin and Harriet Feldman...capture creative approaches to teaching evidence-based practice. This book includes comprehensive and unique strategies for teaching evidence-based practice for all types of learners across a variety of educational and clinical practice settings. The concrete examples of teaching assignments provided in the book bring the content alive and serve as a useful, detailed guide for how to incorporate this material into meaningful exercises for learners. Levin and Feldman's book is a truly wonderful, necessary resource for educators working in all healthcare professional programs as well as clinical settings." —From the Foreword by
Bernadette Mazurek Melnyk, PhD, RN, CPNP/NPP, FAAN, FNAP

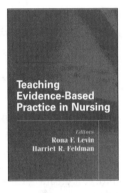

Based on the idea that nursing students and nurses at all levels can contribute to the development of a scientific base for nursing practice by critiquing and questioning guidelines, treatments, and outcomes of their own practice, this book examines the ways in which the teaching and learning of evidence-based practice (EBP) occurs. The book provides useful strategies for educators and facilitates the work of faculty to develop curricula that incorporate EBP and the work of nurses implementing EBP in the clinical setting.

Partial Contents

Part I: Setting the Stage

Part II: The Basics of Teaching/Learning Evidence-Based Practice

Part III: Teaching/Learning Evidence-Based Practice in the Academic Setting

Part IV: Teaching/Learning Evidence-Based Practice in the Clinical Setting

2006   400pp   0-8261-3155-7   softcover

11 West 42nd Street, New York, NY 10036-8002 • Fax: 212-941-7842
Order Toll-Free: 877-687-7476 • Order On-line: www.springerpub.com

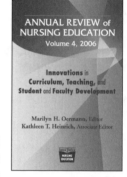